Advances in Laparoscopy and Minimally Invasive Surgery

Guest Editor

MICHAEL P. TRAYNOR, MD, MPH

OBSTETRICS AND GYNECOLOGY CLINICS OF NORTH AMERICA

www.obgyn.theclinics.com

Consulting Editor
WILLIAM F. RAYBURN, MD, MBA

December 2011 • Volume 38 • Number 4

SAUNDERS an imprint of ELSEVIER, Inc.

W.B. SAUNDERS COMPANY
A Division of Elsevier Inc.

Elsevier, Inc. • 1600 John F. Kennedy Blvd. • Suite 1800 • Philadelphia, PA 19103-2899

http://www.theclinics.com

OBSTETRICS AND GYNECOLOGY CLINICS OF NORTH AMERICA Volume 38, Number 4
December 2011 ISSN 0889-8545, ISBN-13: 978-1-4557-0475-0

Editor: Stephanie Donley

Obstetrics and Gynecology Clinics (ISSN 0889-8545) is published quarterly by Elsevier Inc., 360 Park Avenue South, New York, NY 10010-1710. Months of issue are March, June, September, and December. Periodicals postage paid at New York, NY, and additional mailing offices. Subscription price per year is $293.00 (US individuals), $498.00 (US institutions), $146.00 (US students), $3353.00 (Canadian individuals), $628.00 (Canadian institutions), $214.00 (Canadian students), $428.00 (foreign individuals), $628.00 (foreign institutions), and $214.00 (foreign students). To receive student/ resident rate, orders must be accompanied by name of affiliated institution, date of term, and the signature of program/ residency coordinator on institution letterhead. Orders will be billed at individual rate until proof of status is received. Foreign air speed delivery is included in all *Clinics* subscription prices. All prices are subject to change without notice. POSTMASTER: Send address changes to *Obstetrics and Gynecology Clinics*, Elsevier Health Sciences Division, Subscription Customer Service, 3251 Riverport Lane, Maryland Heights, MO 63043. **Customer Service: Telephone: 1-800-654-2452 (U.S. and Canada); 314-447-8871 (outside U.S. and Canada). Fax: 314-447-8029. E-mail: journalscustomerservice-usa@elsevier.com (for print support); journalsonlinesupport-usa@ elsevier.com (for online support).**

Reprints. For copies of 100 or more of articles in this publication, please contact the Commercial Reprints Department, Elsevier Inc., 360 Park Avenue South, New York, New York 10010-1710. Tel.: 212-633-3818; Fax: 212-462-1935; E-mail: reprints@elsevier.com.

Obstetrics and Gynecology Clinics of North America is also published in Spanish by McGraw-Hill Interamericana Editores S.A., P.O. Box 5-237, 06500, Mexico; in Portuguese by Reichmann and Affonso Editores, Rio de Janeiro, Brazil; and in Greek by Paschalidis Medical Publications, Athens, Greece.

Obstetrics and Gynecology Clinics of North America is covered in *MEDLINE/PubMed (Index Medicus)*, *Excerpta Medica, Current Concepts/Clinical Medicine, Science Citation Index, BIOSIS, CINAHL,* and *ISI/BIOMED.*

Printed and bound by CPI Group (UK) Ltd, Croydon, CR0 4YY
Transferred to Digital Print 2011

GOAL STATEMENT

The goal of *Obstetrics and Gynecology Clinics of North America* is to keep practicing physicians up to date with current clinical practice in OB/GYN by providing timely articles reviewing the state of the art in patient care.

ACCREDITATION

The *Obstetrics and Gynecology Clinics of North America* is planned and implemented in accordance with the Essential Areas and Policies of the Accreditation Council for Continuing Medical Education (ACCME) through the joint sponsorship of the University of Virginia School of Medicine and Elsevier. The University of Virginia School of Medicine is accredited by the ACCME to provide continuing medical education for physicians.

The University of Virginia School of Medicine designates this enduring material activity for a maximum of 15 *AMA PRA Category 1 Credit*(s)™ for each issue, 60 credits per year. Physicians should only claim credit commensurate with the extent of their participation in the activity.

The American Medical Association has determined that physicians not licensed in the US who participate in this CME enduring material activity are eligible for a maximum of 15 *AMA PRA Category 1 Credit*(s)™ for each issue, 60 credits per year.

Credit can be earned by reading the text material, taking the CME examination online at http://www.theclinics.com/home/cme, and completing the evaluation. After taking the test, you will be required to review any and all incorrect answers. Following completion of the test and evaluation, your credit will be awarded and you may print your certificate.

FACULTY DISCLOSURE/CONFLICT OF INTEREST

The University of Virginia School of Medicine, as an ACCME accredited provider, endorses and strives to comply with the Accreditation Council for Continuing Medical Education (ACCME) Standards of Commercial Support, Commonwealth of Virginia statutes, University of Virginia policies and procedures, and associated federal and private regulations and guidelines on the need for disclosure and monitoring of proprietary and financial interests that may affect the scientific integrity and balance of content delivered in continuing medical education activities under our auspices.

The University of Virginia School of Medicine requires that all CME activities accredited through this institution be developed independently and be scientifically rigorous, balanced and objective in the presentation/discussion of its content, theories and practices.

All authors/editors participating in an accredited CME activity are expected to disclose to the readers relevant financial relationships with commercial entities occurring within the past 12 months (such as grants or research support, employee, consultant, stock holder, member of speakers bureau, etc.). The University of Virginia School of Medicine will employ appropriate mechanisms to resolve potential conflicts of interest to maintain the standards of fair and balanced education to the reader. Questions about specific strategies can be directed to the Office of Continuing Medical Education, University of Virginia School of Medicine, Charlottesville, Virginia.

The faculty and staff of the University of Virginia Office of Continuing Medical Education have no financial affiliations to disclose.

The authors/editors listed below have identified no professional or financial affiliations for themselves or their spouse/partner:
Shan Biscette, MD; Jennifer Cho, MD; Sarah L. Cohen, MD; Babak Hajhosseini, MD; Carla Holloway, (Acquisitions Editor); William Irvin, MD (Test Author); Louise P. King, MD, JD; Charles R. Rardin, MD; William F. Rayburn, MD, MBA (Consulting Editor); Robert M. Rogers, Jr., MD; Richard H. Taylor, MD; Michael P. Traynor, MD (Guest Editor); and Jennie Yoost, MD.

The authors/editors listed below identified the following professional or financial affiliations for themselves or their spouse/partner:
Andrew I. Brill, MD is on the Speakers' Bureau and is on the Advisory Board for Karl Storz, Ethicon, and Conceptus, and is on the Speakers' Bureau for Smith & Nephew.
Jon I. Einarsson, MD, MPH is a consultant for Ethicon Endo-Surgery.
Stuart Hart, MD is a consultant and is on the Speakers' Bureau for Covidien, Stryker, and Boston Scientific.
Paige Hertwick, MD is an industry funded research/investigator and is on the Speakers' Bureau for Merck Pharmaceutical Corp.
Fred M. Howard, MS, MD is a consultant for Ethicon Womens Health & Urology, and is on the Speakers' bureau for Abbott Laboratories and Ortho Womens Health & Urology.
Malcolm G. Munro, MD, FRCS(C) is a consultant for Boston Scientific, Inc., Conceptus, Inc., Ethicon Womens Health and urology, Karl Storz Endoscopy Americas, and Bayer Health Care; and, is on the Speakers' Bureau for Ethicon Endosourgery.
Camran Nezhat, MD is an industry funded research/investigator for Storz, Covidien, Plasma Jet, Intuitive Surgical, and J&J, and owns stock with Aragon Surgical and Avantis.
Farr Nezhat, MD receives speaking honorarium from Genzyme and Plasma Surgical.
Jonathan Reinstine, MD receives research funding and is on the Speakers' Bureau for Merck Pharmaceutical.
Marshall L. Smith, MD, PhD owns stock in Patton Surgical, and is employed by KASM Designs.
Craig Sobolewski, MD is a consultant for Covidien and TransEnterix, is on the Speakers' Bureau for Covidien, owns stock with TransEnterix, and is on the Adviosry Board for Carefusion.
Patrick P. Yeung, Jr., MD is a consultant for Covidien and Lumenis, and is on the Speakers' Bureau for Covidien.

Disclosure of Discussion of non-FDA approved uses for pharmaceutical products and/or medical devices:

The University of Virginia School of Medicine, as an ACCME provider, requires that all faculty presenters identify and disclose any off-label uses for pharmaceutical and medical device products. The University of Virginia School of Medicine recommends that each physician fully review all the available data on new products or procedures prior to clinical use.

TO ENROLL

To enroll in the Obstetrics and Gynecology Clinics of North America Continuing Medical Education program, call customer service at 1-800-654-2452 or visit us online at www.theclinics.com/home/cme. The CME program is available to subscribers for an additional fee of $180.00

Contributors

CONSULTING EDITOR

WILLIAM F. RAYBURN, MD, MBA
Randolph Seligman Professor and Chair, Department of Obstetrics and Gynecology;
Chief of Staff, University Hospital, University of New Mexico Health Science Center,
Albuquerque, New Mexico

GUEST EDITOR

MICHAEL P. TRAYNOR, MD, MPH
Kaiser Sunnyside Medical Center, Clackamas, Oregon

AUTHORS

SHAN BISCETTE, MD, FACOG
Fellow of Operative Gynecologic Endoscopy, Department of Obstetrics, Gynecology
and Women's Health, University of Louisville School of Medicine, Louisville, Kentucky

ANDREW I. BRILL, MD
Director of Minimally Invasive Gynecology, California Pacific Medical Center, San
Francisco, California

JENNIFER CHO, MD
Department of Obstetrics & Gynecology, North Shore University Hospital, Manhasset,
New York

SARAH L. COHEN, MD
Division of Minimally Invasive Gynecologic Surgery, the Department of Obstetrics and
Gynecology, Brigham and Women's Hospital, Boston, Massachusetts

JON I. EINARSSON, MD, MPH
Division of Minimally Invasive Gynecologic Surgery, the Department of Obstetrics and
Gynecology, Brigham and Women's Hospital, Boston, Massachusetts

BABAK HAJHOSSEINI, MD
Center for Special Minimally Invasive and Robotic Surgery, Department of Obstetrics
and Gynecology, Stanford University, Palo Alto, California

STUART HART, MD
University of South Florida, Tampa, Florida

PAIGE HERTWECK, MD
Director, Pediatric and Adolescent Gynecology Fellowship; Chief of Gynecology, Kosair
Children's Hospital, Louisville, Kentucky

FRED M. HOWARD, MS, MD
Professor Emeritus and Associate Chair of Obstetrics and Gynecology, University of
Rochester School of Medicine and Dentistry, Rochester, New York; Chairman of the
Board, International Pelvic Pain Society, Schaumburg, Illinois

LOUISE P. KING, MD, JD
Center for Special Minimally Invasive and Robotic Surgery, Department of Obstetrics and Gynecology, Stanford University, Palo Alto, California

MALCOLM G. MUNRO, MD, FACOG, FRCS(c)
Professor, Department of Obstetrics & Gynecology, David Geffen School of Medicine at University of California, Los Angeles; Director of Gynecologic Services, Kaiser Permanente, Los Angeles Medical Center, Los Angeles, California

CAMRAN NEZHAT, MD, FACOG
Center for Special Minimally Invasive and Robotic Surgery, Departments of Obstetrics, Gynecology and Surgery, Stanford University, Palo Alto, California

FARR NEZHAT, MD, FACOG
Division of Gynecologic Oncology, St Luke-Roosevelt Hospital and Columbia University, New York, New York

CHARLES R. RARDIN, MD
Associate Professor, Obstetrics and Gynecology, Alpert Medical School of Brown University; Director, Fellowship Program in Female Pelvic Medicine and Reconstructive Surgery; Director, Robotic and Laparoscopic Surgery, Women & Infants Hospital, Providence, Rhode Island

JONATHAN REINSTINE, MD
Clinical Professor, Department of Obstetrics, Gynecology and Women's Health, University of Louisville School of Medicine, Louisville, Kentucky

ROBERT M. ROGERS JR, MD
Northwest Women's Health Care, Kalispell, Montana

MARSHALL L. SMITH, MD, PhD
Medical Director, Clinical Education and Innovation, Banner Health, Phoenix; Clinical Professor, Department of Obstetrics & Gynecology, University of Arizona, Tucson; Adjunct Clinical Professor, Biomedical Informatics, Arizona State University, Phoenix, Arizona

CRAIG SOBOLEWSKI, MD
Duke University Medical Center, Durham, North Carolina

RICHARD H. TAYLOR, MD
Northwest Women's Health Care, Kalispell, Montana

PATRICK P. YEUNG JR, MD
Saint Louis University, St Louis, Missouri

JENNIE YOOST, MD
Fellow, Pediatric and Adolescent Gynecology, Kosair Children's Hospital, Louisville, Kentucky

Contents

Although not a new concept, recent advances in surgical instrumentation have resulted in a renewed interest in the single-puncture approach to a variety of gynecologic procedures. These advances include novel designs for port systems, articulating instrumentation, and flexible laparoscopes. Herein, we describe strategies for overcoming the traditional obstacles associated with utilizing multiple instruments via a single incision to triangulate to a target. These obstacles include external instrument clashing and internal "sword fighting." Evidence that supports a potential benefit to this approach is also described.

Gynecologic laparoscopy has gained momentum in the past 2 decades. It is considered the standard of care in the treatment of certain pathology in the pediatric and adolescent populations such as endometriosis, ovarian cystectomy, ovarian torsion, and ovarian transposition. The application of laparoscopy in pregnancy, however, has been slow to gain widespread acceptance. Physiologic and anatomic changes in the pregnant patient introduce certain risks unique to this population. Although pregnancy is considered a relative contraindication for laparoscopic procedures, data indicate that these concerns may be unwarranted when procedures are performed by skilled surgeons. Appendicitis, cholecystitis, ovarian torsion, and symptomatic adnexal masses are some of the more common conditions necessitating intervention. Although prospective studies of laparoscopic surgery in pregnancy are lacking, there are numerous case reports affirming the feasibility of this approach.

The competent gynecologic surgeon has a sure, working knowledge of the anatomy in the field of pelvic dissection and is expert in the techniques and in the "millimeter by millimeter" progression of surgical dissections. When operating in the pelvis, several questions arise: "In what anatomic area am I dissecting?" defines the anatomy to be dissected out. "What dissection techniques will I use here?" gives the surgeon the confidence to proceed with the operation, while safeguarding the integrity of the surrounding anatomic structures. With less blood loss and less trauma, the surgeon may expect a better patient outcome.

THE CLINICS ARE NOW AVAILABLE ONLINE!

Access your subscription at:
www.theclinics.com

Foreword

Advances in the knowledge and technical skills in laparoscopy and minimally invasive surgery support the need for a special issue dedicated to this subject in *Obstetrics and Gynecology Clinics of North America*. The discipline of gynecology has changed in the past decades, with the emergence of specialties with fellowship training requirements in advanced laparoscopy. In addition, special interest groups have organized to form societies dedicated to advances in laparoscopy, minimally invasive surgery, and office procedures.

The practice of gynecology was less complicated 25 years ago when surgical options were more invasive. Now, an explosion in medical and surgical knowledge has led an impetus for change. Many consider changes, such as robotic surgery, to be symbols of scientific progress within gynecology, while others view these changes as being part of a retrogressive super specialization that is ongoing in medical education. Regardless of those perspectives, these changes have challenged the clinical practice and surgical competence of many gynecology surgeons.

Mastering the variety of surgical approaches to clinical problems within a field as broad as gynecology can be formidable. To make certain that the broadest source of information is available, the authors in this issue discuss such disorders as uterine leimyomata, adnexal masses, and endometriosis that can be amenable to minimally invasive surgery. This requires drawing from a knowledge base to procure and filter through clinical and laboratory data to make a rational surgical treatment plan. An effort was also made in this issue to present a balanced view of the more significant complications that influence surgical outcomes.

To gain skills in advanced laparoscopy and minimally invasive surgery, the clinician is best guided and instructed by experienced teachers and accomplished surgeons and inspired toward self-directed learning. Clearly, there is no replacement for experience in the surgical suite. Unfortunately, many recent resident graduates and younger obstetrician-gynecologists have neither encountered the diversity of clinical situations nor dealt with the more unusual surgical complications to feel comfortable. As described in many of the articles, a learning alternative is through carefully crafted simulations designed to stimulate the decision-making and surgical approach. To achieve that goal, the authors constructed a series of clinical vignettes to teach diagnosis, therapy, and surgical alternatives.

An article on pelvic anatomy was written to coordinate the relationships of the female pelvis with the technical aspects of the various minimally invasive surgical procedures. A more complete understanding of the muscular, vascular, and neurological relationships of the pelvic viscera is emphasized as a prerequisite for successful outcomes in pelvic surgery. This functional description of anatomy cites important areas of the pelvis where operative injuries occur to the nearby urinary tract and bowel.

It is our desire that this issue will inspire and activate attention to issues of pelvic surgery from an array of experienced gynecologic surgeons. On behalf of these knowledgeable contributors, I hope that the practical information provided herein will

Obstet Gynecol Clin N Am 38 (2011) xi–xii
doi:10.1016/j.ogc.2011.10.002
0889-8545/11/$ – see front matter © 2011 Elsevier Inc. All rights reserved.

obgyn.theclinics.com

aid in the implementing of well-planned approaches to women requiring laparoscopy or minimally invasive surgery.

William F. Rayburn, MD, MBA
Department of Obstetrics and Gynecology
University of New Mexico School of Medicine
MSC10 5580; 1 University of New Mexico
Albuquerque, NM 87131-0001, USA

E-mail address:
wrayburn@salud.unm.edu

Minimally Invasive Urogynecology

Charles R. Rardin, MD[a,b,c,]*

KEYWORDS

- Pelvic floor defects • Minimally invasive • Laparoscopy
- Urogynecology • Sacrocolpopexy

The term "minimally invasive" generally represents the efforts on the part of the surgeon to reduce the impact of surgery on the patient, both in terms of incision burden, as well patient discomfort and recovery of normal health status. The recognition of the importance of these characteristics has pervaded all aspects of surgery—there is widespread acceptance of the role of minimization of incision size, use of self-retaining retractors, and other measures to improve the patients' overall experience and recovery, and these might be considered efforts to reduce the invasiveness of surgery in general, even laparotomy. There is more at stake than short term discomfort, cosmesis, and return to activities, though; a growing body of evidence suggests that, at least in some populations such as the obese or those with malignancies, laparoscopic surgery can confer added safety to the patient by minimizing complications associated with larger incision, and significantly reduced intraoperative blood loss.

The advent of laparoscopy for gynecologic surgery was greeted with much enthusiasm; the potential advantages in decreased postoperative pain,[1] rapid recuperation,[2] decreased adhesion formation,[3] and preferable cosmetic result led to a rapid increase in the rate of tubal ligation. The usefulness of the laparoscope as a diagnostic tool was quickly realized, and it enjoyed popularity in the diagnosis and treatment of chronic pelvic pain and endometriosis, as well as in surgical sterilization.

As the tool of the laparoscope has been applied to more advanced surgical procedures, these advantages to the patient have remained significant, and other advantages were realized. The microscopic visualization of the laparoscope has improved identification and avoidance of the vascular structures that have compli-

The author has nothing to disclose.

[a] Department of Obstetrics and Gynecology, Alpert Medical School of Brown University, Box G-A1, Providence, RI 02912, USA

[b] Fellowship Program in Female Pelvic Medicine and Reconstructive Surgery, Women & Infants Hospital, 101 Dudley Street, Providence, RI 02905, USA

[c] Robotic and Laparoscopic Surgery, Women & Infants Hospital, 101 Dudley Street, Providence, RI 02905, USA

* Corresponding author. 695 Eddy Street, Suite 12, Providence, RI 02903.

E-mail address: crardin@wihri.org

Obstet Gynecol Clin N Am 38 (2011) 639–649

doi:10.1016/j.ogc.2011.09.001

0889-8545/11/$ – see front matter © 2011 Elsevier Inc. All rights reserved.

obgyn.theclinics.com

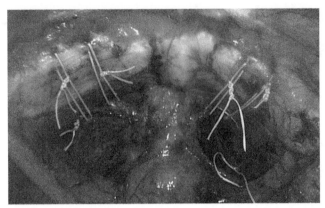

Fig. 1. Laparoscopic burch procedure. Permanent suture is used to support the vaginal fibromuscularis, at the levels of the midurethra and the urethrovesical junction, to Cooper's ligament, providing support to the bladder neck while avoiding overcorrection. When a transperitoneal approach is used, the supravesical peritoneal incision should be closed to avoid complications.

cated retropubic procedures. Additionally, the pneumoperitoneum used during laparoscopy provided some measure of tamponade, again reducing the nuisance of venous oozing during the retropubic dissections. Finally, patient satisfaction with the laparoscopic approach to urogynecologic procedures is favorable.[4]

LAPAROSCOPIC PELVIC RECONSTRUCTIVE SURGERY TECHNIQUES
Laparoscopic Burch Colposuspension Procedure

The retropubic colposuspension, along with suburethral slings, has become, to many, the gold standard for treatment of urodynamic stress incontinence due to bladder neck hypermobility without intrinsic sphincter deficiency.[5] The Burch procedure or, more accurately, the Tanagho modification of the Burch procedure,[6] was performed laparoscopically and described by Vancaillie in1991,[7] with publication of a case series soon afterward.[8,9] The laparoscopic advantages of visualization, hemostasis, and quick recovery for the generally healthy population helped to make this a popular procedure for adaptation to the laparoscopic approach. Some reports suggested higher failure rates when the procedure was significantly altered (eg, using mesh-and-staple techniques, or using a single suture on each side instead of 2)[10]; this underlines the importance of preserving technique when adopting a laparoscopic approach. The most recent iteration of the Cochrane Database of Systematic Reviews concludes that when 2 paravaginal sutures are used on each side, data suggest that laparoscopic Burch is equivalent to open Burch in terms of efficacy at 2 years and preferable in terms of pain, complications, and hospitalization.[11]

Technique

Similar to the open technique, the laparoscopic Burch procedure involves retropubic dissection, clearing of the paraurethral and paravesical fascia, and placement of 2 sutures on each side (one at the urethrovesical junction, the other at the midurethra, at least 2 cm lateral to the urethra itself), which are then suspended from Cooper's ligament ipsilaterally (**Fig. 1**). Suture placement in the paraurethral tissue is facilitated by elevating the tissue with the surgeon's finger in the vagina. Practitioners vary widely in their techniques of assessing the right amount of bladder neck elevation; however, the data have shown that correction of hypermobility is a requirement for successful outcome.[12] Overcorrection, though, can lead to voiding dysfunction; therefore, suture bridges are left to prevent overcorrection. It is also advisable to close any peritoneal incision to prevent incarceration of bowel within these suture bridges.

With the popularity of minimally- invasive slings, the popularity of the Burch procedure has waned; the skillset required and operative time tend to favor the newer generations of slings, and success rates of these slings are at least as high, or, in some series, higher. [13] Interest in the Burch procedure was regenerated, to some degree, by the CARE trial, in which patients undergoing open sacrocolpopexy for vaginal vault prolapse were randomized to receive, or not receive, a concomitant Burch procedure, regardless of preoperative urodynamic findings.[14] Patients who underwent the Burch procedure were half as likely to report postoperative stress incontinence as their counterparts. Many practitioners who have developed skills in laparoscopic prolapse repair procedures offer laparoscopic Burch colposuspension in light of these findings.

Laparoscopic Cystocele (Paravaginal Defect) Repair

Although the traditional repair of cystocele (colporrhaphy) has involved the cen- tral plication of the pubocervical connective tissue, the idea that anterior compartment defects can be lateral (paravaginal), as well as central, was first published nearly a century ago.[15] As the surgical reattachment of anterior vaginal fibromuscularis (sometimes, if erroneously, known as "pubocervical fascia") to the arcus tendineus of the fasciae pelvis (or "white line" of the pelvic sidewall) is more challenging than simple colporrhaphy, this idea lay dormant until the 1970s, when Richardson postulated that the majority of cystoceles are a result of this lateral disruption.[16] More recent anatomic studies have confirmed that lateral defects are usually present in cases of anterior compartment prolapse and bladder neck hypermobility.[17] Biomechanical modeling studies confirm the hypothesis that paravaginal support defects, as well as apical defects, may be required in the development of cystoceles.[18] It stands to reason that a central repair for a lateral defect may reasonably be expected to yield suboptimal success rates, and 1- to 2-year anatomic success rates of 80% to 90% have been observed.[19,20]

Technique

The laparoscopic paravaginal repair, as with the Burch procedure, starts with retrograde filling of the bladder, supravesical peritoneal incision, and dissection of the retropubic space. As the goal is the reattachment along the full length of arcus tendineus along the pelvic sidewall, the dissection must be carried out more laterally than is required for the Burch. For this reason, the peritoneal incision is usually taken beyond the medial umbilical folds; care must be taken to avoid injury to the inferior epigastric vessels. Similarly, identification and protection of the obturator neurovascular bundles is crucial.

After the paravesical vaginal tissue is cleared with gentle dissection, a series of permanent sutures is used to reattach this tissue to the obturator internus muscle on each side (**Fig. 2**). The appearance of the arcus tendineus along the sidewall may be variable; one study showed that the condensation of fibers known as the "white line" are often avulsed and thus attached to the paravaginal fascia, rather than intact along the pelvic sidewall. Thus the surgeon may not always have the clear visual cue along the sidewall. Whether the arcus is readily visible, its original location between the ischial spine and the inferior edge of the pubic ramus can be located by palpation

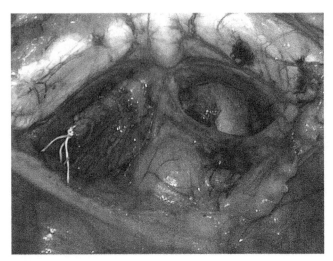

Fig. 2. Laparoscopic paravaginal defect repair. Permanent sutures are used to reapproximate the anterolateral vaginal sulcus to the arcus tendineus fasciae pelvis. Note the complete paravaginal detachment on the right side, with partial repair completed on the left side.

under laparoscopic observation. The surgeon will appreciate the fact that, in this approach, the tissues being sutured together are adjacent; in the vaginal paravaginal repair, the vaginal sutures must be placed with the tissue everted, and thus distant from the targeted area of reattachment.

Laparoscopic Repair of Vault Prolapse: Uterosacral Ligament Suspension

Many variations of uterosacral ligament vault suspension has been described vaginally and are variously known as uterosacral suspensions, culdeplasties, or McCall procedures; several extensive series provide support for the popularity of these procedures.[21] The abdominal or laparoscopic approaches are also feasible; whatever the approach, the technique involves identifying the intact remnants of the utero- sacral ligaments, at or above the level of the ischial spines, which are then sutured to the ipsilateral aspects of the posterior and anterior fibromuscularis of the vaginal vault. It should be noted that, in the case of tissue attenuation, an enterocele sac is likely to be found between these intact anterior and posterior layers of fibromuscularis. The vaginal approach can be made difficult by the challenge of identifying the proximal ligament remnants. In addition, the suture, if permanent (as many advise), must be tied extraluminally, which can be difficult; alternatively, an absorbable suture can be tied within the vaginal lumen. The possibility of ureteral compromise necessitates the use of intraoperative cystoscopy. The visualization of the ureters throughout their pelvic course that laparoscopy can provide may be an additional benefit.

Technique

Laparoscopic uterosacral vault suspension can be performed at the time of hyster- ectomy, or remotely from hysterectomy, in the case of vaginal vault prolapse. After the ureters and the rectum are identified, the uterosacral ligaments are identified at the level of the ischial spines. Permanent suture is then brought through the ligaments at this level; tensiometry studies have demonstrated that laparoscopically placed sutures in the uterosacral ligaments have as much tensile strength as vaginally placed sutures.[22] With the proximal uterosacral ligament thus captured, the sutures are then brought ipsilaterally through the full thickness of the posterior and anterior vaginal walls (excluding epithelium) at the cuff. The attenuated enterocele sac that may lie at the apex, between anterior and posterior vaginal tissue planes, can often be visualized with the use of the vaginal probe. Some surgeons advocate the excision of this attenuated tissue sac; whether or not it is removed, the supporting sutures should be placed beyond it, on the intact fasciae. Advocates of this procedure point out that it is restorative of the original anatomic support and vaginal axis.

The vaginal uterosacral vault suspension, at the time of or remote from vaginal hysterectomy, enjoys popularity as a method of vault suspension, and is variously known as a "high" or "deep" uterosacral suspension, or McCall's culdeplasty. Even advocates, however, acknowledge that preserving ureteral safety during this procedure can be a challenge; one series observed a ureteral compromise rate of 11%.[23] In contrast, the laparoscopic approach may afford enhanced visualization of the ureter, and the ability to dissect and capture the proximal uterosacral ligament more completely; in one series comparing vaginal repairs (McCall with anterior repair) with laparoscopic repairs (uterosacral vault suspension with paravaginal defect repair) at the time of vaginal hysterectomy observed a reduction of ureteral compromise from nearly 5% to zero, with improved anatomic outcomes in both the apical and anterior compartments.[24]

Sacrocolpopexy

The uterosacral vault suspension procedure described relies on the presence and identification of useful uterosacral remnants; it also depends on vaginal sutures at the vault apex for long-term success. In addition, for the reasons outlined earlier, the vaginal apex, in the presence of an enterocele, may represent the most attenuated segment of the entire vagina. Vaginal techniques of vault suspension, including the vaginal version of the uterosacral vault suspension, as well as the sacrospinous ligament fixation, may be susceptible to the same vulnerability. For these reasons, many surgeons prefer the sacrocolpopexy using permanent materials. Although not anatomic in the strictest sense, it has been shown to yield a vaginal axis that is closer to normal than that found after vaginal sacrospinous ligament fixation.[25] It also permits the placement of multiple suture points along the anterior and posterior vaginal walls, distributing tension over a wider area and decreasing the likelihood of suture pullout. In its abdominal version, it has been demonstrated to have a remarkably low recurrence rate over the long term. It is considered by many to be the most definitive repair for vault prolapse, with published anatomic success rates of 78% to 100%.[26]

Technique

A peritoneal incision over the sacral promontory is made and the underlying anterior longitudinal ligament of the sacrum is visualized. Laparoscopically, the pneumoperitoneum facilitates dissection of the retroperitoneal adipose and areolar tissue, and the microscopic visualization allows easier identification of the sacral vessels which, if injured, can retract into the sacrum and results in catastrophic bleeding. It should be noted, however, that the left common iliac vein, which lies just below and inferior to its arterial counterpart, can be compressed by the pneumoperitoneum, and therefore inadvertently injured. For this reason, the dissection over the sacral promontory should be kept slightly to the right of the midline. This incision is carried down into the pelvis, remaining slightly to the right of midline (to avoid mesenteric vasculature) but well medial to the right ureter. This incision allows for the retroperitonealization of the mesh after the suspension; alternatively, the peritoneum can be tunneled rather than opened entirely.

After the vaginal vault is prepared by dissecting peritoneum off of the anterior and posterior aspects (and the development of the vesicovaginal and rectovaginal spaces, respectively), a permanent synthetic graft is affixed to both sides of the vaginal vault. At that point, the mesh (either formed in the shape of a Y, or with 2 separate pieces of mesh) is affixed directly to the anterior longitudinal ligament of the sacrum, with a series of permanent sutures. Care should be taken to avoid or preemptively coagulate the middle sacral vessels, and tools to control for pre-sacral bleeding, such as hemostatic agents and the ability to apply directed pressure, should always be readily available. Many practitioners recommend that the peritoneum be closed over the graft to reduce the likelihood of bowel incarceration or adhesion, though little comparative data exist to support this view.

Multiple retrospective reports support the benefits of minimally invasive techniques in the execution of this form of vaginal support. As has been demonstrated in many other arenas, laparoscopic sacrocolpopexy in the hands of trained surgeons yields similar efficacy while enhancing hemostasis and reducing postoperative pain and hospitalization,[27] while preserving anatomic success rates.[28,29] Here, as before, the principle that laparoscopy is a means of access, and that the steps of the procedures should be identical to that of the open technique, are of utmost importance.

OTHER RECONSTRUCTIVE PROCEDURES
Rectocele

Variations on the above procedures have been performed and described for the treatment of similar conditions. Laparoscopic rectocele repair has been described, in a procedure that involves the extended dissection of the rectovaginal septum all the way to the perineal body, and either plicating the levator musculature[30] or suturing mesh material in place.[31] Similarly, some surgeons advocate the advancement of the posterior dissection and mesh fixation during sacrocolpopexy down to the level of the perineal body in order to address defects in the rectovaginal septum. In principle, this approach to mesh-based repair of the posterior wall may enhance outcomes by eliminating vaginal incisions, which are thought to be contributory in the development of problematic mesh erosion. It should be noted that, with more aggressive dissection of the posterior vaginal wall, the importance of identification of the rectum with a probe is that much greater.

Uterine Preservation

In addition, several studies have called into question the practice of routine extirpation of prolapsed uteri.[32,33] Patients interested in uterine preservation value the availability of this choice, and the elimination of the hysterectomy decreases blood loss, hospitalization, and other complications.[34] Clearly, patients must understand that future pregnancy and delivery may have deleterious effects on the repair, cervical surveillance remains necessary, and hysterectomy may be needed in the future. This option continues to be valued by some women and some practitioners. Both the uterosacral ligament suspension (**Fig. 3**), and the sacrocolpopexy using mesh, can be performed for the treatment of uterine prolapse among women who desire uterine conservation; the techniques are very similar to those described for vault prolapse earlier.

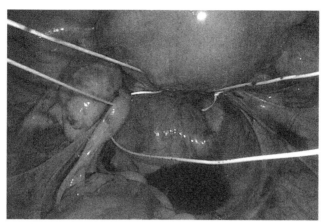

Fig. 3. Laparoscopic uterosacral uterine suspension. Permanent sutures are used to approximate the proximal uterosacral ligament portion to the distal insertion on the upper vagina and cervix ipsilaterally. The ureters and rectum are visualized prior to suture placement. Some surgeons opt to perform a culdoplasty as well.

ROBOTICS IN PELVIC RECONSTRUCTIVE SURGERY

The da Vinci robotic surgical platform (Intuitive Surgical, Sunnyvale, CA, USA) represents a significant technical advancement in the instrumentation for laparoscopic surgery. Sitting at a console, the surgeon uses controls to operate a set of robotic arms fitted with specialized instruments. The main advantages include motion scaling (converting large movements of the surgeon to very fine movements of the instruments), instruments with an additional degree of motion (known as an endowrist), and the enhancement of dexterity and psychomotor performance (through tremor-stabilizing algorithms). The da Vinci system also uses binocular, 3- dimensional video, enhancing depth perception.The performance of these systems in the training of residents is in the early stages. One study demonstrated a steeper (ie, more rapid) learning curve, among both experienced and inexperienced surgeons, in the performance of drills using a robotic system.[35] Another study demonstrated that laparoscopic drills were completed more quickly with the robotic system compared to traditional laparoscopy and that novice surgeons on the robot performed as quickly, and in some cases more quickly, than expert surgeons with traditional laparoscopy.[36]

The continued refinement of these systems may redress some of the deficiencies in laparoscopic training by improving skill acquisition. While there is continued debate about whether robotic assistance is required, there is little doubt that the advent of the robotic platform has increased the availability of minimally invasive sacrocolpopexy. Although prospective comparative trials comparing traditional to robotic sacrocolpopexy are not yet available, there are data that suggest that, compared to abdominal sacrocolpopexy, the robotic approach takes longer in the operating room but patients benefit with less blood loss and shorter length of stay and short-term anatomic outcomes that are as good or better.[37]

OTHER FORMS OF MINIMALLY INVASIVE UROGYNECOLOGY
Minimally Invasive Suburethral Slings

The trocar-based Tension-free Vaginal Tape (TVT) suburethral sling procedure heralded the arrival of a new paradigm of reconstructive surgery, and the principles underlying its effectiveness continue to be applied to new pelvic reconstructive techniques. There are 3 important ways in which the TVT (Ethicon, Sommerville, NJ, USA) differs from the slings that preceded it: midurethal placement (rather than at the bladder neck), trocar-based delivery, performed blindly and with minimal dissection, and self-retaining mesh that required no additional fixation. A variety of tensioning techniques exist, with the key provision that, at rest, the tape should exert no tension on the underside of the urethra. The blind passage of trocars through the retropubic space requires advanced anatomic understanding and confidence on the part of the surgeon and is beset with a certain incidence of bladder perforation and, much less commonly, bowel and vascular injury.

Taking several principles of the TVT, de Leval introduced the transobturator tape (TOT) sling in 2003. It is similar to the TVT in its trocar-based, midurethral placement, and self-retaining mesh materials. However, this technique passes the trocar through the obturator membrane avoiding entry into the true pelvis. This lateral approach seeks to reduce the likelihood of injury to pelvic organs or vasculature. A large-scale, multicenter, randomized trial with nearly 600 patients observed efficacy equivalence between these sling types. Tradeoffs were seen in other parameters; voiding dysfunction requiring reoperation was required in 2.7% of retropubic sling patients, compared to none in the TOT group, whereas neurologic complications (most commonly, leg or thigh pain) was higher in the TOT group.[38]

One important caveat is that many comparative trials between retropubic and transobturator midurethral slings excluded patients with intrinsic sphincter deficiency (ISD, variably defined, but generally including low measures of abdominal leak point pressures, maximum urethral closure pressures, or both). A randomized trial comparing these 2 slings in a population of women with ISD found that the risk of failure and need for repeat surgery was 2.6 times higher among patients receiving a transobturator sling.[39]

Limitations to the popularity of laparoscopic urogynecology have included the perception of increased difficulty, prolonged operative times, a protracted learning curve, and a relative paucity of advanced pelvic reconstructive training centers nationally. In addition, specific laparoscopic CPT code sets for reconstructive surgery have been largely inaccurate or lacking entirely, and reimbursement levels have not provided an incentive for surgeons to adopt minimally invasive techniques.

More recently, the advent of vaginal mesh–based prolapse repair techniques and device kits have offered the promise of a new age in minimally invasive pelvic reconstructive surgery. Early iterations of these devices used extrapelvic trocars to pass extensions of mesh through the levator musculature and pelvic sidewalls. More recent versions have focused the main point of focus on the sacrospinous ligament. Advocates of transvaginal mesh procedures point to decreased operative times and the avoidance of entry into the peritoneal cavity as significant benefits. A large number of case series, cohorts, and some comparative trials have confirmed the feasibility of such approaches; data are accumulating that support the use of synthetic mesh in the anterior compartment through a vaginal incision.[40] However, such techniques have also introduced a new wave of complications. The MAUDE database (1,000 entries to which triggered the October 2008 FDA Public Health Notification about vaginal mesh) reports, in recent years, a 3:1 ratio of complications from mesh kits compared to the much more commonly performed sling procedures.[41] Mesh kits appear to have the highest rate of reoperation for complications of apical suspension procedures, while traditional vaginal surgeries for apical support have the highest reoperation for failure rates.[42] These issues have helped to reinvigorate interest in the abdominal or laparoscopic approaches to mesh reconstruction, in which mesh complication rates appear to be lower (although quality comparative studies in this regard are lacking).

SUMMARY

Laparoscopic and other forms of minimally invasive pelvic floor defect repair represent alternative approaches to performing established procedures; laparoscopy can offer benefits to the surgeon (improved visualization, access for multiple procedures) and patient (decreased pain, scar formation, recuperation, and improved cosmesis). Many practitioners prefer the term "minimal access surgery" to the more prevalent "minimally invasive surgery," as, ideally, only the route of access, not the procedure itself, is changed. Similarly, dialogue and debate about the merits and concerns of trocar-based mesh prolapse repair kits continue. While gynecology will benefit from further investigations of outcomes of minimally invasive pelvic reconstruction, there is evidence already that these techniques are feasible and offer options and advantages in the treatment of patients with pelvic floor disorders.

REFERENCES

1. Brumsted J, Kessler C, Gibson C, et al. A comparison of laparoscopy and laparotomy for the treatment of ectopic pregnancy. Obstet Gynecol 1988;71:889–92.
2. Azziz R, Steinkampf MP, Murphy A. Postoperative recuperation: relation to the extent of endoscopic surgery. Fertil Steril 1989;51:1061–4.
3. Filmar S, Gomel V, McComb PF. Operative laparoscopy versus open abdominal surgery: a comparative study on postoperative adhesion formation in the rat model. Fertil Steril 1987;48:486–9.
4. Myers DL, Peipert JF, Rosenblatt PL, et al. Patient satisfaction with laparoscopic Burch retropubic urethropexy. J Reprod Med 2000;45:939–43.
5. Leach GE, Dmochowski RR, Appell RA, et al. Female Stress Urinary Incontinence Clinical Guidelines Panel summary report on surgical management of female stress urinary incontinence. The American Urological Association. J Urol 1997; 158:875–80.
6. Tanagho EA. Colpocystourethropexy; the way we do it. J Urol 1976;116:751.
7. Vancaillie TG, Schuessler W. Laparoscopic bladderneck suspension. J Laparoendosc Surg 1991;1:169–73.
8. Albala DM, Schuessler WW, Vancaillie TG. Laparoscopic bladder suspension for the treatment of stress incontinence. Semin Urol 1992;10:222–6.
9. Liu CY, Paek W. Laparoscopic retropubic colposuspension (Burch procedure). J Am Assoc Gynecol Laparosc 1993;1:31–5.
10. Persson J, Teleman P, Eten-Bergquist C, et al. Cost-analyses based on a prospective, randomised study comparing laparoscopic colposuspension with tension-free vaginal tape procedure. Acta Obstet Gynecol Scand 2002;81:1066–73.
11. Dean N, Ellis G, Herbison GP, et al. Laparoscopic colposuspension for urinary incontinence in women. Cochrane Database Syst Rev 2006;3:CD002239.
12. Zivkovic F, Tamussino K. Mechanism of postoperative urinary incontinence. Int Urogynecol J 2001 12:199–202.
13. Paraiso MF, Walters MD, Karram MM, et al. Laparoscopic Burch colposuspension versus tension-free vaginal tape: a randomized trial.Obstet Gynecol 2004;104:1249–58.
14. Brubaker L, Cundiff G, Fine P, et al. Abdominal sacrocolpopexy with Burch colposuspension to reduce urinary stress incontinence. N Engl J Med 2006;354:1557–66.
15. White GR. An anatomic operation for the cure of cystocele. Am J Obstet Dis Woman Child 1912;56:286–90.

16. Richardson AC, Lyon JB, Williams NL. A new look at pelvic relaxation. Am J Obstet Gynecol 1976;126:568.
17. Delancey JO. Fascial and muscular abnormalities in women with urethral hypermobility and anterior vaginal wall prolapse. Am J Obstet Gynecol 2002;187:93–8.
18. Chen L, Ashton-Miller JA, DeLancey JO. A 3D finite element model of anterior wall support to evaluate mechanisms underlying cystocele formation. J Biomech 2009; 42:1371–7.
19. Seman EI, Cook JR, O'Shea RT. Two-year experience with laparoscopic pelvic floor repair. J Am Assoc Gynecol Laparosc 2003;10:38–45.
20. Benhia-Willison F, Seman EI, Cook JR, et al. Laparoscopic paravaginal repair of anterior compartment prolapse. J Minim Invasive Gynecol 2007;14:475–80.
21. Shull BL, Bachofen C, Coates KW, et al. A transvaginal approach to repair of apical and other associated sites of pelvic organ prolapse with uterosacral ligaments. Am J Obstet Gynecol 2000;183:1365–73.
22. Culligan PJ, Miklos JR, Murphy M, et al. The tensile strength of uterosacral ligament sutures: a comparison of vaginal and laparoscopic techniques. Obstet Gynecol 2003;101:500–3.
23. Barber MD, Visco AG, Weidner AC, et al. Bilateral uterosacral vaginal vault suspension with site-specific endopelvic fascia defect repair for treatment of pelvic organ prolapse. Am J Obstet Gynecol 2000;183:1402–10.
24. Rardin CR, Erekson EA, Sung VW, et al. Uterosacral colpopexy at the time of vaginal hysterectomy: comparison of laparoscopic and vaginal approaches. J Reprod Med 2008;54:273–80.
25. Sze EH, Meranus J, Kohli N, et al. Vaginal configuration on MRI after abdominal sacrocolpopexy and sacrospinous ligament suspension. Int Urogynecol J Pelvic Floor Dysfunct 2001;12:375–9.
26. Nygaard IE, McCreery R, Brubaker L, et al. Abdominal sacrocolpopexy: a comprehensive review. Obstet Gynecol 2004;104:805–23.
27. Hsiao KC, Latchamsetty K, Govier FE, et al. Comparison of laparoscopic and abdominal sacrocolpopexy for the treatment of vaginal vault prolapse. J Endourol 2007;21:926–30.
28. Paraiso MF, Walters MD, Rackley RR, et al. Laparoscopic and abdominal sacral colpopexies: a comparative cohort study. Am J Obstet Gynecol 2005;192:1752–8.
29. Klauschie JL, Suozzi BA, O'Brien MM, et al. A comparison of laparoscopic and abdominal sacral colpopexy: objective outcome and perioperative differences. Int Urogynecol J Pelvic Floor Dysfunct 2009;20:273–9.
30. Ross JW. Techniques of laparoscopic repair of total vault eversion after hysterectomyJ Am Assoc Gynecol Laparosc 1997;4:173–83.
31. Lyons TL, Winer WK. Laparoscopic rectocele repair using polyglactin mesh. J Am Assoc Gynecol Laparosc 1997;4:381–4.
32. Hefni M, El-Toukhy T, Bhaumik J, et al. Sacrospinous cervicocolpopexy with uterine conservation for uterovaginal prolapse in elderly women: an evolving concept. Am J Obstet Gynecol 2003;188:645–50.
33. Barranger E, Fritel X, Pigne A. Abdominal sacrohysteropexy in young women with uterovaginal prolapse: long-term follow-up. Am J Obstet Gynecol 2003;189:1245–50.
34. Diwan A, Rardin CR, Strohsnitter WC, et al. Laparoscopic uterosacral ligament uterine suspension compared with vaginal hysterectomy with vaginal vault suspension for uterovaginal prolapse. Int Urogynecol J Pelvic Floor Dysfunct 2006;17:79–83.
35. Prasad SM, Maniar HS, Soper NJ, et al. The effect of robotic assistance on learning curves for basic laparoscopic skills. Am J Surg 2002;183:702–7.

36. Sarle R, Tewari A, Shrivastava A, et al. Surgical robotics and laparoscopic training drills. J Endourol 2004;18:63–6.
37. Geller EJ, Siddiqui NY, Wu JM, et al. Short-term outcomes of robotic sacrocolpopexy compared with abdominal sacrocolpopexy. Obstet Gynecol 2008;112:1201–6.
38. Richter HE, Albo ME, Zyczynski HM, et al. Retropubic versus transobturator midurethral slings for stress incontinence. N Engl J Med 2010;362:2066–76.
39. Schierlitz L, Dwyer PL, Rosamilla A, et al. Effectiveness of tension-free vaginal tape compared with transobturator tape in women with stress urinary incontinence and intrinsic sphincter deficiency: a randomized controlled trial. Obstet Gynecol 2008;112:1253–61.
40. Murphy M, for the Society of Gynecologic Surgeons Systematic Review Group. Clinical practice guidelines on vaginal graft from the Society of Gynecologic Surgeons. Obstet Gynecol 2008;112:1123–30.
41. Mucowski SJ. Use of vaginal mesh in the face of recent FDA warnings and litigation. Am J Obstet Gynecol 2010;203:e1–4.
42. Diwadkar GB, Barber MD, Feiner B. Complication and reoperation rates after apical vaginal prolapse surgical repair: a systematic review. Obstet Gynecol 2009;113:1377.

Total and Supracervical Hysterectomy

Sarah L. Cohen, MD, Jon I. Einarsson, MD, MPH*

KEYWORDS

- Laparoscopy • Hysterectomy • Supracervical
- Postoperative care

The first successful vaginal hysterectomy was performed in 1813 by Conrad Langenbeck, followed 40 years later by the first abdominal hysterectomy.[1,2] It was not until the work of laparoscopic surgical pioneers Kurt Semm and Harry Reich in the late 1980s, however, that a significant procedural transformation occurred with the introduction of laparoscopic hysterectomy.[3,4] Hysterectomy surveillance data reveal that nearly 600,000 hysterectomies are performed in the United States annually, with nearly a quarter of US women undergoing the procedure by the time they reach age 60.[5,6] As of 2005, the most common benign indications for hysterectomy include uterine leiomyomas (41%), endometriosis (18%), and prolapse (15%).[7] Other frequent indications are chronic pelvic pain and abnormal uterine bleeding, although indications for hysterectomy vary widely depending on demographic characteristics. As hysterectomy is the most common non–pregnancy-related surgical procedure among women, it is critical to continually evaluate best practice recommendations.

According to a 2005 query of national databases, the rates of approach to hysterectomy were distributed as follows: 64% abdominal, 22% vaginal, and 14% laparoscopic.[8] In addition to clinical characteristics, socioeconomic variables were also found to be predictors of surgical route, with underserved populations being less likely to undergo laparoscopy. The 2009 Cochrane meta-analysis regarding optimal route for hysterectomy reports that patients who underwent laparoscopic hysterectomy demonstrated a more rapid return to normal activity, less postoperative pain, fewer infectious/febrile episodes, smaller drop in hemoglobin, earlier discharge from the hospital, and improved quality of life at both 6 and 16 weeks postoperatively.[9] Alternatively, laparoscopic hysterectomy held no advantage when evaluated against vaginal hysterectomy. Compared to abdominal and vaginal approaches, disadvantages that have been attributed to laparoscopy included longer operative time and increased rate of urinary tract injuries. The Cochrane meta-analysis, however, was

Dr Einarsson is a consultant for Ethicon Endo-Surgery. The authors have nothing to disclose.
Division of Minimally Invasive Gynecologic Surgery, the Department of Obstetrics and Gynecology, Brigham and Women's Hospital, 75 Francis Street, ASB 1-3, Boston, MA 02115, USA
* Corresponding author.
E-mail address: jeinarsson@partners.org

Obstet Gynecol Clin N Am 38 (2011) 651–661
doi:10.1016/j.ogc.2011.09.002
0889-8545/11/$ – see front matter © 2011 Elsevier Inc. All rights reserved.

underpowered to detect a significant difference in rates of urinary tract injury and much of the data regarding such injuries were derived from nonrandomized trials. There is also emerging data supporting the superiority of laparoscopic hysterectomy over vaginal hysterectomy with regard to postoperative pain, blood loss, and duration of hospital stay.[10,11]

The American College of Obstetricians and Gynecologists guidelines state that laparoscopic hysterectomy should be the approach of choice when vaginal hysterectomy is not feasible, for example in cases with significant extrauterine pathology, a narrow pelvic arch or vagina, undescended or immobile uterus, nulliparity, prior cesarean delivery, or enlarged uterus.[12] The American Association of Gynecologic Laparoscopists (AAGL) further asserts that factors such as obesity or prior cesarean delivery should not preclude a laparoscopic approach.[13] The AAGL goes on to define the rare true contraindications to laparoscopic hysterectomy: patients with significant cardiopulmonary disease who are unable to tolerate increased intraperitoneal pressure, cases of malignancy where morcellation would be required, severely distorted anatomy, and lack of access to appropriately trained surgeons or facilities.

PREOPERATIVE PLANNING

In addition to a thorough history and physical exam, the preoperative work-up for hysterectomy includes imaging of the pelvis as appropriate and exclusion of genital tract malignancy. Recent Pap smear data should be reviewed, and patients with risk factors for endometrial hyperplasia/malignancy, including obesity, postmenopausal bleeding, and anovulatory bleeding over the age of 35, should be advised to have endometrial sampling prior to surgery.[14] This is particularly important if the surgical plan will involve morcellation of tissue specimen. Although useful in evaluating endometrial neoplasia, endometrial biopsy and curettage share a low predictive value in the case of uterine sarcomas, failing to detect approximately a third of cases.[15] In cases where the preoperative diagnosis was leiomyomata, incidental finding of leiomyosarcoma has been reported in 0.5% of cases.[16] Patients with concerning clinical symptoms such as rapid uterine growth or postmenopausal fibroid symptoms may benefit from magnetic resonance imaging and/or serum lactate dehydrogenase measurements in an effort to distinguish between degenerating leiomyoma and sarcoma.[17]

During the preoperative planning phase, it is also important to hold an informed discussion with patients regarding risks specific to laparoscopic hysterectomy, including visceral or vascular injury and conversion to laparotomy. Published incidences of complications include the following ranges obtained from large trials and surgical registries: conversion to laparotomy 2.7% to 3.9%, urologic injury 1.2% to 3%, bowel injury 0.2% to 0.4%, and hemorrhage 2% to 5.1%.[18–20] Safety of laparoscopic hysterectomy in the obese patient population has also been demonstrated.[21] Two caveats to this discussion are worth mentioning: first, much of the existing data may be outdated and thereby overestimate the incidence of complications due to the rapid advances in surgical technique and evolution of advanced minimally invasive gynecology. Second, it is important for each surgeon to review specific complication rates in his or her individual practice as these may vary greatly with experience or level of case difficulty. For example, one retrospective review of over 1500 laparoscopic hysterectomies found that the risk of bladder injury decreased with surgeon experience and plateaued at 0.4% after 100 cases were performed.[22] This highlights the importance of individualized risk discussions based on surgeon experience and patient characteristics.

After the decision is made regarding the laparoscopic route of hysterectomy, patients should be informed of the option regarding cervical retention or removal. In the early decades of the 20th century, the majority of hysterectomies were completed supracervically. The transition to total hysterectomy by the 1950s was largely motivated by a desire to decrease rates of cervical cancer, as the rate of carcinoma in the residual cervical stump was as high as 1% to 2%.[23] As cervical cancer screening methods advanced, the supracervical approach regained recognition with its proposed advantages in pelvic support and sexual satisfaction. These theoretic advantages of supracervical hysterectomy have not been supported by randomized clinical trials, however.[24–26] Additionally, the 2006 Cochrane review of total versus subtotal hysterectomy concluded that existing data do not support any difference in sexual, bladder, or bowel function between the 2 approaches.[27]

The American College of Obstetricians and Gynecologists cautions that there is a lack of data to support superiority of supracervical hysterectomy and urges practitioners to carefully screen patients for cervical or uterine neoplasia prior to recommending this approach.[28] Should a patient meet criteria and elect to retain her cervix, she should be informed of the need for continued routine cervical cancer screening following hysterectomy. A further concern regarding retention of the cervix is posthysterectomy cyclic bleeding, which has been reported in 11% to 17% of cases.[29,30] Despite these issues, the supracervical procedure may allow for a shorter procedure with less blood loss and faster immediate postoperative recovery.[27,31] Additionally, one must consider the risk of vaginal cuff dehiscence or cellulitis when total hysterectomy is performed. Although the risk of vaginal vault dehiscence is low, it has been described more commonly following laparoscopic hysterectomy with a reported incidence of up to 1.2%.[32] It has been hypothesized that the higher risk of dehiscence observed with laparoscopic cases may result from energy sources used to create the colpotomy, differences with suturing techniques, or the fact that patients return to baseline activities and intercourse earlier. In practice, it may be advisable to counsel patients with history of cervical neoplasia or significant pain symptoms toward removal of the cervix; alternately, patients with predominantly bulk or bleeding symptoms may be good candidates for consideration of a supracervical approach. **Table 1** summarizes a recommended strategy regarding patient counseling for total or supracervical hysterectomy.

OPERATIVE APPROACH

A successful laparoscopic procedure begins with proper patient positioning to maximize anatomic access, prevent perioperative neuropathy, and ensure ergonomic stance for the surgeon. The patient should be placed in dorsal lithotomy position using booted stirrups with majority of weight placed on the heels, moderate flexion at

Table 1 Recommendations for type of hysterectomy			
	Recommended Type of Hysterectomy		
Clinical Features	Total Hysterectomy	Supracervical Hysterectomy	Either
History of cervical dysplasia	X		
Endometriosis/pelvic pain or dyspareunia	X		
Plan concomitant apical prolpase repair with mesh		X	
Abnormal uterine bleeding/fibroids			X

the knee and hip, and minimal abduction and external rotation at the hip in order to avoid sciatic and femoral nerve damage.[33,34] Care should also be taken to avoid excess compression of the lateral fibular head against the lower extremity stirrups, using padding as necessary to avoid damage to the common peroneal nerve. Bilateral arms should be tucked at the patient's side in neutral position with hand flat against lateral thigh and appropriate protection of the wrist and fingers from compression; padding of the posteromedial aspect of the elbow is recommended as well to avoid ulnar neuropathy. Traction devices such as egg-crate foam or vacuum-beanbag mattress should be used to prevent the patient from slipping toward the head of the bed while in Trendelenberg position. Factors specific to gynecologic surgery that are known to increase the risk for intraoperative nerve injury include improper or prolonged (longer than 4 hours) lithotomy position and the use of shoulder braces.[33] At the beginning of the procedure, the operating table is placed in level position at the lowest table height with a video monitor directly facing each surgeon to facilitate operator comfort.

Although some surgeons prefer not to use a uterine manipulator system at the time of laparoscopic hysterectomy, the authors have found that a uterine manipulator can be valuable in order to facilitate mobilization of the uterus, ensure cephalad displacement at the time of colpotomy, delineate of the vaginal cuff, and maintain pneumoperitoneum. Two commonly used systems include the RUMIUterine Manipulator (Cooper-Surgical, Trumbull, CT, USA) and the VCare Uterine Manipulator/Elevator (ConMed Endosurgery, Utica, NY, USA). The RUMI uterine manipulator is superior at demarcating the vaginal fornices, especially in the setting of a long cervix, although placement of this manipulator is a multistep process that can be time-consuming.[35] Conversely, the VCare manipulator is a less-bulky and easier-to-insert device and may be particularly useful in the patients with a narrow introitus. Foley catheter is also inserted into the bladder to continuous straight drainage at the time of uterine manipulator placement.

A variety of abdominal entry techniques may be used as dictated by surgeon comfort and preference, including closed Veres needle entry, direct trocar entry, or open Hasson-style peritoneal access. The initial step of peritoneal access can be one of the most dangerous steps in the operation, accounting for 40% to 50% of complications and carrying a risk of vascular injury of 0.9 in 1000 cases and bowel injury of 1.8 in 1000 cases.[36,37] The 2008 Cochrane meta-analysis on laparoscopic entry concluded that there is no evidence for superiority of any one technique, though the included studies were small and potentially underpowered to assess safety differentials. In cases of suspected intra-abdominal adhesive disease, history of umbilical hernia, large uteri extending above the umbilicus, or failed initial entry at the umbilical location, an initial left upper quadrant entry at Palmer's point is recommended. For multiport laparoscopic hysterectomy, the authors typically use a 10/12-mm trocar at the umbilicus in addition to 2 (for supracervical hysterectomy) or 3 (total hysterectomy) 5-mm accessory trocars. The bilateral lower quadrant trocars are placed under direct visualization lateral to the rectus abdominis muscles, 2 cm superior and 2 cm medial to the anterior superior iliac spine. Additionally, the fourth trocar is placed approximately 8 cm superior and parallel to the lower left trocar site, approximately along the same horizontal plane as the umbilicus. Preferences for trocar positioning vary widely by provider; however, in cases involving laparoscopic suturing, the authors find the left-sided ipsilateral suturing position (2 parallel accessory trocars on the left side of the patient) to be ergonomically superior.

A solid understanding of electrosurgical principles is crucial to safe laparoscopic hysterectomy. Options for energy sources include monopolar electrosurgery, bipolar electrosurgery, and vessel sealing/ligation devices. Monopolar electrosurgery can create a cutting, fulgurating, and desiccating effect, though it may be more prone to hazards such as direct or capacitive coupling and insulation failure.[38] Bipolar electrosurgery does not share the same risks of visceral injury as monopoloar energy, although it is characterized by longer time to coagulation, char formation, and lateral thermal spread. Advanced vessel sealing/ligation disposable devices that may be useful in laparoscopic hysterectomy include LigaSure sealing device (Covidien, Boulder, CO, USA), PlaskmaKinetics (PK) Sealer (Gyrus ACMI Medical, Maple Grove, MN, USA), Harmonic Scalpel (Ethicon Endo-Surgery, Somerville, NJ, USA), and EnSeal Vessel Fusion System (SurgRx, Palo Alto, CA, USA). These advanced vessel sealing devices are differentiated by varying degrees of lateral thermal spread, burst pressure, smoke creation, and speed of vessel sealing.[39] With appropriate knowledge of device-specific characteristics and principles of electrosurgery, any of the above-mentioned options can be safely used. The authors' preference is to use an HarmonicScalpel along with a reusable bipolar grasper for vessel sealing and dissection. In our experience, this combination allows for precise dissection and adhesiolysis capability as well as the capability to obtain secure hemostasis even in the setting of large vascular pedicles. Additionally, we strongly prefer using only one disposable energy source from a cost-savings standpoint.

After visual inspection of the abdomen and pelvis and performing adhesiolysis as necessary, the procedure is begun by addressing the adnexa. The authors recommend a technique of remaining close to the ovary when dividing the infundibolopelvic or utero-ovarian ligament in order to avoid ascending uterine vasculature (if conserving ovaries) or pelvic sidewall structures (if removing ovaries)[35] (**Fig. 1**). As the round ligament is transected, care is taken to avoid engorged parametrial venous plexus if present, and the anterior and posterior leaves of the broad ligament are opened (**Fig. 2**). The dissection is continued anteriorly to develop the incision along the vesicouterine peritoneum, and the correct areolar plane is identified with care to avoid any perivesical fat, which indicates proximity to the bladder (**Fig. 3**). The uterine vasculature is skeletonized and dessicated at the level of the internal cervical os; during this phase, the uterus is elevated cephalad with the manipulator in order to increase the distance of uterine vessels from the ureter (**Fig. 4**). It may be advisable

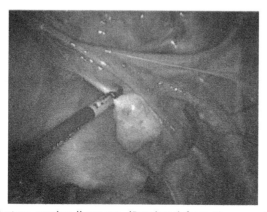

Fig. 1. Control of utero-ovarian ligament. (*Reprinted from* Einarsson JI, Suzuki Y. Total laparoscopic hysterectomy: 10 steps toward a successful procedure. Rev Obstet Gynecol 2009;2:57–64; with permission.)

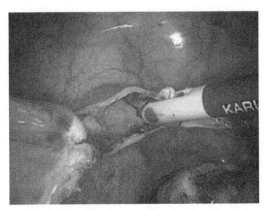

Fig. 2. Dissection of broad ligament. (*Reprinted from* Einarsson JI, Suzuki Y. Total laparoscopic hysterectomy: 10 steps toward a successful procedure. Rev Obstet Gynecol 2009;2:57–64; with permission.)

to dessicate the uterine vasculature bilaterally before incising the pedicle, particularly in cases of large uteri or when concern for increased blood loss exists. The vascular pedicle is created relatively high and mobilized laterally in further effort to avoid ureteral injury and create a clearly delineated vascular bundle that can be safely controlled in the event of future bleeding (**Fig. 5**).

In the case of laparoscopic supracervical hysterectomy, the uterus is transected at the level of the internal os; this may be accomplished with the Harmonic Scalpel or monopolar devices such as a spatula, scissor, or loop. When using the Harmonic Scalpel, it is useful to use the "drill-in" method, where the harmonic is activated on the mex setting and then drilled into the cervix, followed by closure of the clamp, which facilitates the transaction of the cervix. Following transaction, the cervical stump is carefully inspected for hemostasis and the endocervical canal is dessicated in an effort to decrease risk of postoperative cyclic bleeding. Morcellation is then accomplished using a mechanical tissue morcellator device.

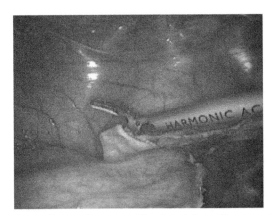

Fig. 3. Opening vesicouterine peritoneum. (*Reprinted from* Einarsson JI, Suzuki Y. Total laparoscopic hysterectomy: 10 steps toward a successful procedure. Rev Obstet Gynecol 2009;2:57–64; with permission.)

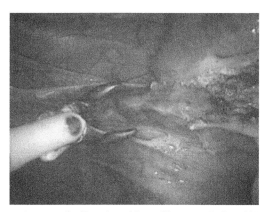

Fig. 4. Dessicating uterine vessels. (*Reprinted from* Einarsson JI, Suzuki Y. Total laparoscopic hysterectomy: 10 steps toward a successful procedure. Rev Obstet Gynecol 2009;2:57–64; with permission.)

When total laparoscpic hysterectomy is performed, the vaginal fornices are identified with continued cephalad pressure on the uterine manipulator. Once the bladder is sufficiently mobilized inferiorly, the colpotomy is made in a circumferential fashion using either the Harmonic Scalpel, monopolar spatula, or scissors (**Fig. 6**). When using a monopolar instrument, it is preferable to use a pure-cut current since this minimized thermal spread, which may help to prevent cuff necrosis and breakdown. The uterus is delivered through the vagina, with laparoscopic or vaginal morcellation performed as indicated by the size of the specimen, and pneumoperitoneum is maintained by occluding the vaginal canal (eg, with the uterus itself, a glove filled with surgical sponges, or a suction bulb). The vaginal cuff may be sutured closed using a variety of techniques and suture types, though the authors typically prefer a single-layer running closure with barbed suture. Regardless of suture choice and decision regarding running or interrupted sutures, care should be taken to ensure

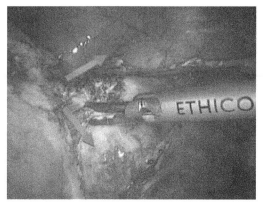

Fig. 5. Lateralizing uterine vascular pedicle. (*Reprinted from* Einarsson JI, Suzuki Y. Total laparoscopic hysterectomy: 10 steps toward a successful procedure. Rev Obstet Gynecol 2009;2:57–64; with permission.)

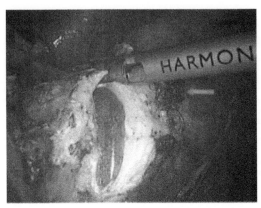

Fig. 6. Colpotomy. (*Reprinted from* Einarsson JI, Suzuki Y. Total laparoscopic hysterectomy: 10 steps toward a successful procedure. Rev Obstet Gynecol 2009;2:57–64; with permission.)

bites of at least 1 cm in thickness are taken that include the vaginal mucosa as well as rectovaginal and pubocervical fascia.

The procedure is complete after all vascular pedicles have been observed for hemostasis; it may be beneficial to lower the intraperitoneal pressure to enhance inspection of bleeding. Abdominal wall fascial defects over 8 to 10 mm are typically sutured closed separately from skin incisions. During the course of the procedure, the anatomic course of the ureter should be identified (including retroperitoneal dissection and ureterolysis if necessary) at key steps including transaction of the infundibulopelvic ligament and creation of uterine vascular pedicles. Although some studies support universal intraoperative cystoscopy for the identification of urinary tract injury at the time of hysterectomy, it is important to realize that a normal cystoscopy does not guarantee lack of injury, particularly in cases of thermal damage.[40,41] We do not use routine cystoscopy in our practice, however employ it liberally when clinically indicated. If a thermal injury to the ureter is suspected, it is important to perform a complete ureterolysis to fully visualize the course of the ureter. A priori ureterolysis is also recommended in certain situations such as severe endometriosis, in severe pelvic adhesive disease, or in patients with a broad ligament or cervical myoma.

POSTOPERATIVE CARE

Unless otherwise indicated by the specific surgical proceedings, the Foley catheter can typically be removed at the end of the laparoscopic hysterectomy case. Early ambulation and oral intake should be encouraged. The decision on whether to discharge the patient on the same day of surgery or to admit for a short inpatient stay is dependent on several factors including the patient's comfort level and availability of caretakers at home, medical comorbidities, and whether any complications were encountered in the case. The safety of discharging patients on the day of surgery for uncomplicated supracervical and total hysterectomies has been well documented.[42–45] In addition, patient preferences were investigated in a randomized trial of day-case vs inpatient laparoscopic supracervical hysterectomy; similar satisfaction rates were found with lower self-reported short-term quality of life in the day surgery group.[46] It is reasonable to infer, therefore, that in an appropriately selected and motivated patient population, same-day discharge for laparoscopic hysterectomy may be safe and well-tolerated.

No evidence-based guidelines exist to support physicians' recommendations for patient activity following hysterectomy. General consensus regarding time for pelvic rest following hysterectomy is typically 4 to 8 weeks (on the longer end of the scale for total hysterectomies). Aside from those general considerations, patients are normally counseled to return to normal activities as soon as their comfort allows. A recovery period of 2 to 4 weeks before resumption of the majority of baseline activities can be expected.[47]

SUMMARY

Despite a long history of success with laparoscopic approach to hysterectomy, the majority of hysterectomies in the United States are currently performed via laparotomy.[48-51] Barriers to the integration of laparoscopic hysterectomy include technological difficulties, inadequate training, low levels of peer support, potential for decreased reimbursement and misconceptions about laparoscopic safety, cost, and technical feasibility.[52-54] With the continual evolution of minimally invasive hysterectomy techniques, now including robotic, single-port, and natural-orifice surgery, it is vital to critically evaluate the literature in an effort to offer patients the most safe and effective treatments. This report aims to summarize the available data surrounding both the total and supracervical laparoscopic hysterectomy and to provide concrete suggestions for maximizing success with these procedures.

REFERENCES

1. Langenbeck CJM. Geschichte einer von mir glucklich verichteten extirpation der ganger gebarmutter. Biblioth Chir Ophth Hanover 1817;1:557.
2. Burnham W. Extirpation of the uterus and ovaries for sarcomatous disease. Nelson's Am Lancet 1854;8:147–51.
3. Semm K. Hysterectomy via laparotomy or pelviscopy. A new CASH method without colpotomy. Geburtshilfe Frauenheilkd 1991;51:996–1003.
4. Reich H, de Cripo J, McGlynn F. Laparoscopic hysterectomy. J Gynecol Surg 1989;5:213–5.
5. Merrill RM. Hysterectomy surveillance in the United States, 1997 through 2005. Med Sci Monit 2008;14:CR24–31.
6. Lepine LA, Hillis SD, Marchbanks PA, et al. Hysterectomy surveillance: United States, 1980–1993. MMWR CDC Surveill Summ 1997;46:1–15.
7. Whiteman MK, Hillis SD, Jamieson DJ, et al. Inpatient hysterectomy surveillance in the United States, 2000–2004. Am J Obstet Gynecol 2008;198:e1–34.
8. Jacoby VL, Autry A, Jacobson G, et al. Nationwide use of laparoscopic hysterectomy compared with abdominal and vaginal approaches. Obstet Gynecol 2009;114:1041–8.
9. Nieboer TE, Johnson N, Lethaby A, et al. Surgical approach to hysterectomy for benign gynaecological disease. Cochrane Database Syst Rev 2009;3:CD003677.
10. Candiani M, Izzo S, Bulfoni A, et al. Laparoscopic vs vaginal hysterectomy for benign pathology. Am J Obstet Gynecol 2009;200:e1–7.
11. Ghezzi F, Uccella S, Cromi A, et al. Postoperative pain after laparoscopic and vaginal hysterectomy for benign gynecologic disease: a randomized trial. Am J Obstet Gynecol 2010;203:118.e1–8.
12. ACOG Committee Opinion No. 444: choosing the route of hysterectomy for benign disease. Obstet Gynecol 2009;114:1156–8.
13. AAGL Advancing Minimally Invasive Gynecology Worldwide. AAGL position statement: route of hysterectomy to treat benign uterine disease. J Minim Invasive Gynecol 2011;18:1–3.

14. ACOG Committee on Practice Bulletins—Gynecology. American College of Obstetricians and Gynecologists. ACOG practice bulletin No. 14: management of anovulatory bleeding. Int J Gynaecol Obstet 2001;72:263–71.
15. Bansal N, Herzog TJ, Burke W, et al. The utility of preoperative endometrial sampling for the detection of uterine sarcomas. Gynecol Oncol 2008;110:43–8.
16. Leibsohn S, d'Ablaing G, Mishell DR, et al. Leiomyosarcoma in a series of hysterectomies performed for presumed uterine leiomyomas. Am J Obstet Gynecol 1990;162: 968–74.
17. Seki K, Hoshihara T, Nagata I. Leiomyosarcoma of the uterus: ultrasonography and serum lactate dehydrogenase level. Gynecol Obstet Invest 1992;33:114–8.
18. Canis M, Botchorishvili R, Ang C, et al. When is laparotomy needed in hysterectomy for benign uterine disease? J Minim Invasive Gynecol 2008;15:38.
19. Garry R, Fountain J, Brown J, et al. EVALUATE hysterectomy trial: a multicentre randomised trial comparing abdominal, vaginal and laparoscopic methods of hysterectomy. Health Technol Assess 2004;8:1–154.
20. Mäkinen J, Johansson J, Tomas C, et al. Morbidity of 10 110 hysterectomies by type of approach. Hum Reprod 2001;16:1473–8.
21. Chopin N, Malaret JM, Lafay-Pillet MC, et al. Total laparoscopic hysterectomy for benign uterine pathologies: obesity does not increase the risk of complications. Hum Reprod 2009;24:3057–62.
22. Lafay Pillet MC, Leonard F, Chopin N, et al. Incidence and risk factors of bladder injuries during laparoscopic hysterectomy indicated for benign uterine pathologies: a 14.5 years experience in a continuous series of 1501 procedures. Hum Reprod 2009;24:842–9.
23. Scott JR, Sharp HT, Dodson MK, et al. Subtotal hysterectomy in modern gynecology: a decision analysis. Am J Obstet Gynecol 1997;176:1186–92.
24. Thakar R, Ayers S, Clarkson P, et al. Outcomes after total versus subtotal abdominal hysterectomy. N Engl J Med 2002;347:1318–25.
25. Gimbel H, Zobbe V, Andersen BM, et al. Randomised controlled trial of total compared with subtotal hysterectomy with one-year follow up results. BJOG 2003;110: 1088–98.
26. Learman LA, Summitt RL Jr, Varner RE, et al. A randomized comparison of total or supracervical hysterectomy: surgical complications and clinical outcomes. Obstet Gynecol 2003;102:453–62.
27. Lethaby A, Ivanova V, Johnson NP. Total versus subtotal hysterectomy for benign gynaecological conditions. Cochrane Database Syst Rev 2006;2:CD004993.
28. ACOG Committee. Opinion No. 388 November 2007: supracervical hysterectomy. Obstet Gynecol 2007;110:1215–7.
29. Ghomi A, Hantes J, Lotze EC. Incidence of cyclical bleeding after laparoscopic supracervical hysterectomy. J Minim Invasive Gynecol 2005;12:201–5.
30. Okaro EO, Jones KD, Sutton C. Long term outcome following laparoscopic supracervical hysterectomy. BJOG 2001;108:1017–20.
31. Ghomi A, Cohen SL, Chavan N, et al. Laparoscopic-assisted vaginal hysterectomy vs. laparoscopic supracervical hysterectomy for treatment of nonprolapsed uterus. J Minim Invasive Gynecol 2011;18:205–10.
32. Agdi M, Al-Ghafri W, Antolin R, et al. Vaginal vault dehiscence after hysterectomy. J Minin Invasive Gynecol 2009;16:313–7.
33. Irvin W, Andersen W, Taylor P, et al. Minimizing the risk of neurologic injury in gynecologic surgery. Obstet Gynecol 2004;103:374–82.
34. Agostini J, Goasguen N, Mosnie H. Patient positioning in laparoscopic surgery: Tricks and tips. J Visc Surg 2010;147:227–32.

35. Einarsson JI, Suzuki Y. Total laparoscopic hysterectomy: 10 steps toward a successful procedure. Rev Obstet Gynecol 2009;2:57–64.
36. Vellinga TT, De Alwis S, Suzuki Y, et al. Laparoscopic entry: the modified ALWIS method and more. Rev Obstet Gynecol 2009;2:193–8.
37. Ahmad G, Duffy JM, Phillips K, et al. Laparoscopic entry techniques. Cochrane Database Syst Rev 2008;2:CD006583.
38. Advincula AP, Wang K. The evolutionary state of electrosurgery: where are we now? Curr Opin Obstet Gynecol 2008;20:353–8.
39. Newcomb WL, Hope WW, Schmelzer TM, et al. Comparison of blood vessel sealing among new electrosurgical and ultrasonic devices. Surg Endosc 2009;23:90–6.
40. Ibeanu OA, Chesson RR, Echols KT, et al. Urinary tract injury during hysterectomy based on universal cystoscopy. Obstet Gynecol 2009;113:6–10.
41. Vellinga TT, Suzuki Y, Istre O, et al. Anatomic considerations in gynecologic surgery. Rev Obstet Gynecol 2009;2:137–8.
42. Taylor RH. Outpatient laparoscopic hysterectomy with discharge in 4 to 6 hours. J Am Assoc Gynecol Laparosc 1994;1:S35.
43. Thiel J, Gamelin A. Outpatient total laparoscopic hysterectomy. J Am Assoc Gynecol Laparosc 2003;10:481–82.
44. Morrison JE, Jacobs VE. Outpatient laparoscopic hysterectomy in a rural ambulatory surgery centre. J Am Assoc Gynecol Laparosc 2004;11:359–64.
45. Lieng M, Istre O, Langebrekke A, et al. Outpatient laparoscopic supracervical hysterectomy with assistance of the lap loop. J Minim Invasive Gynecol 2005;12:290–4.
46. Kisic-Trope J, Qvigstad E, Ballard K. A randomized trial of day-case vs inpatient laparoscopic supracervical hysterectomy. Am J Obstet Gynecol 2011;204:e1–8.
47. Claerhout F, Deprest J. Laparoscopic hysterectomy for benign diseases. Best Pract Res Clin Obstet Gynaecol 2005;19:357–75.
48. Wu JM, Wechter ME, Geller EJ, et al. Hysterectomy rates in the United States, 2003. Obstet Gynecol 2007;110:1091–5.
49. Wilcox LS, Koonin LM, Pokras R, et al. Hysterectomy in the United States, 1988-1990. Obstet Gynecol 1994;83:549–55.
50. Jacobson GF, Shaber RE, Armstrong MA, et al. Hysterectomy rates for benign indications. Obstet Gynecol 2006;107:1278–83.
51. Babalola EO, Bharucha AE, Schleck CD, et al. Decreasing utilization of hysterectomy: a population-based study in Olmsted County, Minnesota, 1965–2002. Am J Obstet Gynecol 2007;196:214.e1–214.
52. Einarsson JI, Matteson KA, Schulkin J, et al. Minimally invasive hysterectomies: a survey on attitudes and barriers among practicing gynecologists. J Minim Invasive Gynecol 2010;17:167–75.
53. Englund M, Robson S. Why has the acceptance of laparoscopic hysterectomy been slow? Results of an anonymous survey of Australian gynecologists. J Minim Invasive Gynecol 2007;14:724–8.
54. Warren L, Ladapo JA, Borah BJ, et al. Open abdominal versus laparoscopic and vaginal hysterectomy: analysis of a large United States payer measuring quality and cost of care. J Minim Invasive Gynecol 2009;16:581–8.

Laparoscopic Management of Adnexal Masses

Camran Nezhat, MD[a],*, Jennifer Cho, MD[b], Louise P. King, MD, JD[b], Babak Hajhosseini, MD[c], Farr Nezhat, MD[d]

KEYWORDS

- Adnexal mass • Minimally invasive • Cyst
- Ovarian malignancy • Laparoscopy

The discovery of an adnexal mass is a common clinical problem affecting women of all ages. From 5% to 10% of American women will undergo a surgical procedure in their lifetime owing to a suspected ovarian neoplasm and between 13% and 21% of these women will be diagnosed with ovarian cancer.[1]

Thus, although the majority of adnexal masses are benign, the primary goal of diagnostic evaluation is the exclusion of malignancy. Currently, there is no effective way to screen for ovarian malignancy, and the risk rises with increasing age. Ovarian cancer is the leading cause of death from gynecologic cancers and the fifth leading cause of cancer death in women in the United States, with 15,280 deaths annually and a 1.42% lifetime risk of dying from ovarian malignancy.[2,3] The poor rates of survival result from a lack of early warning signals, sensitive screening, or early detection techniques.[4]

Some women with adnexal masses may present with acute torsion or rupture and peritoneal signs requiring immediate surgical intervention; however, the vast majority of adnexal masses are discovered incidentally during imaging or on pelvic exam.[1,5] Adnexal masses discovered incidentally represent a diagnostic and management dilemma.

This review will detail recent advances in diagnosis, treatment, and, importantly, minimally invasive surgical techniques that have the potential to decrease unnecessary morbidity among patients during evaluation of adnexal masses.

The authors have nothing to disclose.
[a] Center for Special Minimally Invasive and Robotic Surgery, Departments of Obstetrics, Gynecology and Surgery, Stanford University, 900 Welch Road, Suite 400, Palo Alto, CA 94304, USA
[b] Department of Obstetrics and Gynecology, North Shore University Hospital, 300 Community Drive, Manhasset, NY 11030, USA
[c] Center for Special Minimally Invasive and Robotic Surgery, Department of Obstetrics and Gynecology, Stanford University, 900 Welch Road, Suite 403, Palo Alto, CA 94304, USA
[d] Division of Gynecologic Oncology, St Luke-Roosevelt Hospital and Columbia University, 425 West 59th Street, Suite 9B, New York, NY 10019, USA
* Corresponding author.
E-mail address: cnezhat@stanford.edu

Obstet Gynecol Clin N Am 38 (2011) 663–676
doi:10.1016/j.ogc.2011.09.003
0889-8545/11/$ – see front matter © 2011 Elsevier Inc. All rights reserved.

obgyn.theclinics.com

DIAGNOSIS

Most adnexal masses arise from the ovary. Nevertheless, the differential diagnosis for any adnexal mass includes differentiation between an "extraovarian mass" (ectopic pregnancy, tuboovarian abscess, peritoneal inclusion cyst, pedunculated fibroid, diverticular abscess, appendiceal abscess/tumor, fallopian tube cancer, inflammatory/malignant bowel disease, and pelvic kidney) and an "ovarian mass" (physiologic cysts, endometrioma, theca lutein cysts, primary neoplasms, and metastatic carcinoma).[6]

The diagnostic evaluation of a woman with an adnexal mass begins with a thorough history and physical examination. Imaging, with or without laboratory studies, is necessary in a majority of cases. The ultimate diagnostic tool is histological examination.[6,7]

History

Special attention should be paid to the patient's family history, characteristics of her pain, and her menstrual history. It has been shown that more severe or more frequent than expected symptoms of recent onset warrant further diagnostic investigation because they are more likely to be associated with malignant ovarian masses.[8] Nulliparity, history of infertility and/or endometriosis, and a family history of breast, ovarian, or colon cancer are considered risk factors for ovarian cancer.[6,9,10] It has also been shown in recent studies that postmenopausal women who use hormone replacement therapy (HRT) are at an increased risk of ovarian cancer.[11–13]

The most important decision point in assessment of malignant potential for an adnexal mass is the stage of a woman's reproductive life. The suspicion for a malignancy is increased in prepubescent (germ cell tumors) and postmenopausal women (epithelial ovarian cancer) while masses in menstruating women are more likely to be gynecologic and most are functional cysts. Postmenopausal patients with adnexal masses undergoing surgical evaluation have an 8% to 45% chance of malignancy, while malignancy has been found in only 7% to 13% of premenopausal women undergoing similar procedures.[14,15] Nulliparous patients have been shown to have a 2- to 3-fold increased risk of ovarian cancer as compared with parous women. Endometriosis has been associated with increased risk of ovarian cancer and malignant transformation has been demonstrated.[16] Among familial risks, approximately 5% to 10% of epithelial ovarian cancers are suspected to be genetically based, a majority of which include BRCA1 and BRCA2 mutations.[1,17]

Physical Examination

The bimanual and rectovaginal examination focus on the size, location, consistency, and mobility of the adnexal mass to help formulate a differential diagnosis. However, these examinations, even when performed in conjunction with a rectal exam and even when performed under anesthesia, have limited utility both for detection and differentiation of an adnexal mass. Detection rates as low as 60% have been reported.[18] The bimanual exam is limited by body habitus and thus detection rates presumably are hampered even further by obesity.[19]

Imaging

Multiple imaging modalities are used in the diagnosis and the differentiation of adnexal masses including ultrasound, magnetic resonance imaging (MRI), computed tomography (CT), and positron emission tomographic (PET) scanning. Transvaginal sonography has emerged as the imaging modality of choice given its widespread availability, tolerability for the patient, and cost-effectiveness.[1,20] A complete ultrasound assessment will include both a transvaginal and an abdominal component so as to fully characterize masses that may be both pelvic and abdominal. The report should include the size and consistency of the mass (cystic, solid, mixed); its location (ovarian, uterine, bowel); whether unilateral versus bilateral; and the presence or absence of certain characteristics that may help determine an individual's risk of malignancy. Characteristics of ovarian cysts that are generally associated with a higher risk for malignancy include increasing size over multiple imaging studies, septations, excrescences, mural nodules, papillary projections, solid components, and the presence of ascites.[21,22] Color Doppler ultrasonography and 3-dimensional sonography with "vascular sampling" of suspicious areas have also been investigated, but further studies are required to fully delineate their utility. Scoring systems, such as the Pelvic Mass Score (PMS) suggested by Rossi and colleagues, and the Risk of Malignancy Index (RMI), can be used to determine the likelihood of malignancy.[23–25] A meta-analysis of various scoring systems revealed a pooled sensitivity and specificity ranging from 86% to 91% and from 68% to 83%, respectively.[1]

Typical findings for certain benign adnexal masses have been described in smaller studies. Endometriomas will consist of a round homogeneous fluid filled mass with low-level echoes.[26,27] Mature teratomas will contain hypoechoic components and multiple small homogeneous interfaces.[28] Hydrosalpinges appear as tubular sonolucent cysts.[29]

Incidental adnexal masses are sometimes found during CT scans for other indications. As with ultrasonography, a CT scan can help identify the size, location, and relationship of the adnexal mass to other organs. However, a CT scan is a less reliable imaging modality compared to ultrasonography and cannot as easily demonstrate the internal characteristics of adnexal masses. CT scans are most useful for assessing the remainder of the abdomen and pelvis when metastatic disease is suspected. By contrast, in select cases when ultrasonographic findings are uncertain, MRI can help further characterize the adnexal mass.[30] MRI is particularly useful in differentiating the origin of nonadnexal pelvic masses. With each of these imaging modalities, certain characteristics can shed clues as to the etiology of the mass (**Table 1**).[30] There is no current role for PET scan in the evaluation of adnexal masses.

Routine screening for ovarian cancer is not currently recommended by any medical organization.[31,32] However, large-scale studies over recent years have demonstrated the feasibility and potential of multimodal screening strategies.[33–35] Given the low prevalence of ovarian cancer in the general population, any successful screening strategy must have both high specificity and sensitivity; in one review, values of greater than 75% and 99.6%, respectively, were suggested.[36] Early reports from the UK Collaborative Trial of Ovarian Cancer Screening have shown that a multimodal approach to screening involving yearly CA-125 with second-line transvaginal ultrasounds has the highest sensitivity (89.4%) and specificity (99.8%).[34] Investigations will continue to determine the optimal screening method, and novel biomarkers likely will serve to increase both sensitivity and specificity in this important preventative measure.

Laboratory Studies

Laboratory tests used during the evaluation of an adnexal mass should include serum markers, complete blood count, serum electrolytes, urinalysis, and fecal occult blood test.

Table 1
Classification of Adnexal masses by imaging features

	No or Few Solid Elements	Some Solid Elements
Cystic Tumors		
Containing serous fluid	Serous cystadenoma	Borderline serous tumor Serous adenofibroma
Containing mucinous fluid	Mucinous cystadenoma	Borderline mucinous tumor Mucinous adenofibroma
Containing blood	Corpus luteum cyst Endometriotic cyst Benign cyst with secondary hemorrhage	Borderline endometrioid tumor Endometrioid adenofibroma Borderline cyst with secondary hemorrhage
Containing lipid	Teratoma (ie, dermoid cyst)	Teratoma (ie, dermoid cyst)
Predominantly Solid Tumors		
Epithelial		
Serous cystadenocarcinoma		
Mucinous cystadenocarcinoma		
Endometrioid cystadenocarcinoma		
Clear cell cystadenocarcinoma		
Brenner tumor: benign, borderline, or malignant		
Germ cell and sex cord stromal		
Granulosa cell tumor		
Thecoma and other sex cord stromal tumors		
Teratoma (ie, dermoid cyst)		
Dysgerminoma		
Yolk sac tumor		
Other		
Fibroma		
Lymphoma		
Metastatic tumors		

Data from Bharwani N, Reznek RH, Rockall AG. Ovarian cancer management: the role of imaging and diagnostic challenges. Eur J Radiol 2011;78:41–51.

CA-125 is a serum marker that is elevated in approximately 80% of women with ovarian cancer. However, although CA-125 is elevated in 90% of women with advanced disease, it is elevated in only 50% of women with stage I disease at the time of diagnosis.[1,2] In addition, CA-125 is a nonspecific marker that can be elevated in many other conditions, including other malignancies such as endometrial cancer and certain pancreatic cancers; benign gynecologic etiologies such as endometriosis, uterine fibroids, and pregnancy; nongynecologic conditions such as gastroenteritis, pancreatitis, cirrhosis, congestive heart failure, liver failure, pleuritis, pneumonia, or pleural effusion of any origin; and in approximately 1% of healthy patients.[6,37] Thus, CA-125 has both poor sensitivity and poor specificity as a screening test for ovarian cancer. Serum CA-125 levels have been demonstrated to be more accurate among a postmenopausal population with a positive predictive value of 98% and a negative predictive value of 72%. In contrast, in premenopausal patients CA-125 levels have a positive predictive value of only 49%.[38] In recent biomarker studies, combined testing of CA-125 and human epididymis 4 (HE4) provided the greatest level of discrimination between adnexal masses that were benign versus malignant.[39] However, combining the markers HE4 and CA-125 does not seem to lead to more accurate detection rates of ovarian malignancy.[40]

Serum human chorionic gonadotropin (hCG) should be obtained in women of reproductive age to rule out pregnancy and, along with other serum markers such as alpha-fetoprotein (AFP) and lactate dehydrogenase (LDH), can be helpful in young women when a germ cell tumor is suspected. Obtaining estradiol, dehydroepiandro-sterone (DHEA), and testosterone levels may be helpful in women suggested to have functional tumors, such as steroid tumors, or if a girl younger than 12 years is being evaluated.

TREATMENT

The primary goal in the evaluation and the treatment of an adnexal mass at any age is to rule out ovarian malignancy. The suspicion for a malignancy is increased in prepubescent (germ cell tumors) and postmenopausal women (epithelial ovarian cancer).

Medical Therapy

Asymptomatic, small, well-characterized adnexal masses may be observed with regular pelvic examinations and radiologic evaluations in premenopausal women. A recent study supports following simple unilocular ovarian cysts in postmenopausal women without intervention.[41] The American College of Obstetrics and Gynecology notes that simple cysts up to 10 cm in diameter are almost universally benign and can be safely followed without intervention, even in postmenopausal patients.[1] Although hormonal contraceptives are often prescribed to suppress ovarian cysts, reviews have concluded that functional cysts will not regress more quickly with estrogen-progestin contraceptive therapy when compared to expectant management.[42] Adnexal masses detected incidentally during routine sonography in pregnancy can also be followed expectantly. The majority are physiologic or benign tumors that will resolve spontaneously.

A surgical approach should be used if growth occurs in these masses, if the patient becomes symptomatic, or if the mass develops more concerning features, such as solid components or papillary projections. Persistant adnexal masses at extremes of age—pubertal and postmenopausal—should be evaluated surgically as the suspicion for malignancy is high. Postmenopausal patients with adnexal masses undergoing surgical evaluation may have up to a 45% chance of malignancy.[14]

Surgical Therapy

Women with cysts larger than 10 cm and those with findings suspicious for malignancy require surgical exploration. In addition to the cyst's sonographic appearance, findings suspicious for malignancy include no change or an increase in size, a highly elevated CA-125 (>200 U/mL), ascites, suspicion of metastatic disease, or a positive family history.[43] Similar studies indicate that a surgical approach should be used if growth occurs in these masses, if the patient becomes symptomatic, or if the mass develops more concerning features, such as solid components or papillary projections.

The traditional surgical approach to adnexal masses has been via laparotomy. However, regardless of the index of suspicion for malignancy, laparoscopic evaluation of adnexal masses is appropriate in the hands of a skilled laparoscopic surgeon. The sequence of events should parallel those implemented in laparotomy: a thorough evaluation of the abdomen and pelvis, peritoneal washings, cystectomy or adnexectomy as indicated, biopsies of suspicious lesions, and frozen section evaluation. **Fig. 1** demonstrates findings on laparoscopy that are concerning for malignancy. The incidence of unsuspected malignancy ranges from 0.4% to 14% in patients undergoing laparoscopic evaluation for adnexal masses.[44]

Surgical therapy for benign appearing lesions

Ovarian cysts. Our group has previously described optimal laparoscopic management of benign ovarian cysts.[45] The major benefit of the laparoscopic approach in the management of any adnexal mass and especially in instances of benign disease is the avoidance of overtreatment and unnecessary laparotomy.

Surgical treatment of benign appearing cyst must follow the protocol described here including cytologic examination of pelvic washings and frozen section. Cyst aspiration alone is not recommended. The pathologic examination of cyst fluid is not adequate to assess for malignancy. From 10% to 65% of cyst aspirates will be interpreted as benign when in fact malignancy is present. Moreover, cyst recurrence is common with simple aspiration.[45]

An ideal ovarian cystectomy will consist of removal of the cyst intact with limited trauma to residual ovarian tissues. With larger cysts, aspiration is appropriate so as to decompress the mass and assist in dissection and excision. If the cyst ruptures, the resulting contamination is greater than if the cyst were opened and aspirated.[45] Methods for aspiration of larger cysts have previously been described.[45] However, teratomas should be removed intact whenever possible. Laparoscopic management of dermoid cysts was reported as early as 1987.[46–49]

Removal of the cyst wall is essential to prevent recurrence. If the cyst wall cannot be identified, the edge of the ovarian incision can be "freshened" with scissors to reveal a clean edge and assist dissection. A key step in complete excision of a cyst and its wall, whether assisted by aspiration or not, is the atraumatic development of the correct plane between the wall and ovarian tissues. This can be more easily accomplished with the use of hydrodissection. An 18- or 20-gauge needle is introduced through an accessory trocar sleeve. Alternatively, a 7.5-in spinal needle can be introduced through the abdominal wall. Dilute vasopressin is injected between the capsule and ovarian cortex creating a plane that is subsequently developed using the suction-irrigator as a blunt probe. After complete removal of the cyst and capsule, the base is irrigated and hemostasis is ensured using the CO_2 laser or bipolar electrocoagulation. If the ovarian edges overlap well, no further repair is necessary. However, in some instances, fine absorbable microfilament suture can be used to bring the

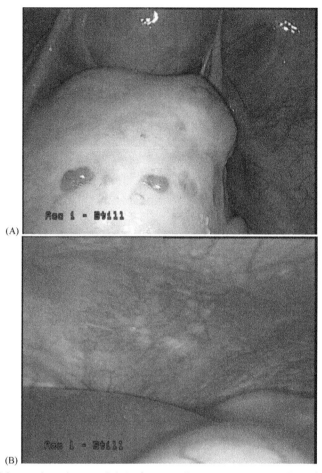

Fig. 1. Suspicious adnexal mass. *(A)* Surface ovarian excrescences positive for malignant implants. *(B)* Metastatic implants visualized during laparoscopic survey in the upper abdomen and anterior abdominal wall.

edges together and promote healing. The sutures should be buried inside the ovary to prevent formation of adhesions.[45]

Excised tissues should be removed with the assist of a specimen removal bag. Methods to aid in removal have been previously described and include further cyst aspiration, morcellation, and decreasing the pneumoperitoneum.[45] The surgeon must ensure that all tissue is removed and that contamination of the anterior abdominal wall does not occur as this can lead to ovarian remnant.

If contamination does occur, for example, if the specimen removal bag ruptures, all efforts must be made to remove all tissue and the incision must be copiously irrigated.

Ovarian remnant. Ovarian remnant syndrome (ORS) is defined as the persistence of functional ovarian tissues after oophorectomy. Laparoscopic management of ovarian remnants was reported as early as 1992.[50,51]

Most women with ORS present with chronic pelvic pain, dyspareunia, and postcoital pain. ORS results from incomplete excision of ovarian tissues at the time of bilateral oophorectomy. A variety of risk factors predispose to this condition and include extensive adhesive disease from endometriosis, pelvic inflammatory disease, inflammatory bowel disease, appendicitis or appendectomy, a history of previous surgeries, and neoplastic lesions.[51]

The sonographic appearance of ovarian remnants varies from small to large and includes both cystic or multiseptated masses with some component of vascularized ovarian tissue. ORS is more likely to occur on the left side because the infundibulopelvic ligament on this side is partially obscured by its relationship to the sigmoid colon and appears shorter leading to incomplete excision.[52] Low or borderline levels of follicle-stimulating hormone in patients with documented bilateral oophorectomy are consistent with the presence of retained ovarian tissue. Clomiphene citrate or human menopausal gonadotropin can be used to increase the remnant's size to aid in the diagnosis preoperatively or to assist in locating the tissue at the time of surgery if extensive adhesions are suspected.

Patients with ORS will have a prior surgical history and the chance of adhesive disease, including anterior abdominal wall adhesions, is likely; thus, an open entry or mapping technique is advised.[51] The surgeon should proceed with extensive and careful retroperitoneal dissection to facilitate identification and removal of all ovarian tissue.

Laparoscopic management of ORS is feasible and safe in the hands of experienced surgeons. Despite objections to the use of minimally invasive approaches in ORS,[53] case series have reported excellent outcomes after laparoscopic management.[50,54–56]

Surgical therapy for probable malignancy

When an obvious epithelial ovarian malignancy is encountered, a complete staging protocol must be performed. This includes complete exploration of the abdomen, total hysterectomy, bilateral salpingo-oophorectomy, omentectomy, pelvic and para-aortic lymph node dissections, biopsies of the undersurface of the right and left diaphragms, and biopsies of the colic gutters followed by a maximal resection of the intra-abdominal tumor. In select cases involving women with limited, early stage, low-grade ovarian cancers, a fertility-sparing procedure may be considered. When malignancy has spread to the abdominopelvic cavity, cytoreduction to minimal or preferably no disease should be performed.

Borderline (low malignant potential) tumors

Borderline ovarian tumors represent 10% to 20% of epithelial ovarian cancers and typically have an excellent prognosis. Survival rates for all borderline ovarian tumors range from 92% among those with advanced stage disease to 98% in those with stage I disease.[57] Borderline ovarian tumors occur predominantly in a premenopausal population with the highest frequency occurring in patients aged 30 to 50; 50% to 85% of these are diagnosed as stage I. The 2 most frequent histologic subtypes of borderline ovarian tumors are serous and mucinous tumors. Serous tumors are bilateral in 30% of cases with concurrent peritoneal implants in 35% of cases.[57] Mucinous tumors are malignant in only 5% of cases with rare case reports of nodal metastases; thus, complete staging may not be necessary in these cases. Appendiceal primaries are quite common among the mucinous tumors, so appendectomy is routinely performed.

Fertility-sparing options in reproductive age patients range from cystectomy to adnexectomy. Recurrence rates vary depending on the surgical approach: adnexectomy recurrence rates range from 0% to 20%, and cystectomy recurrence rates range from 23% to 58%.[57] Laparoscopically assisted hysterectomy for the management of a borderline ovarian tumor was reported in 1992.[58] Since then, laparoscopic staging in borderline ovarian tumors has become increasingly common with advances in endoscopic techniques and instruments.[59]

Early stage invasive ovarian cancer

Early stage invasive ovarian cancer requires complete surgical staging to obtain important prognostic information, to avoid understaging of patients, and to determine the optimal postoperative management. Staging typically includes total abdominal hysterectomy, bilateral salpingo-oophorectomy, omentectomy, peritoneal biopsies, pelvic and para-aortic lymph node dissection, and peritoneal washings. While, traditionally, staging of early ovarian cancer had been performed via laparotomy, there is evidence that, in hands of an experienced laparoscopic surgeon, staging of early ovarian cancer is comparably safe and efficient with similar long-term outcomes.

Advances in laparoscopic management of ovarian malignancy would not have been possible without multiple advances in instrumentation and the introduction of videolaparoscopy.[60–62] Before the introduction of videolaparoscopy, the utility of operative laparoscopy was diminished by two major drawbacks: poor visualization into the intra-abdominal cavity with one eye and the inability of the operative team to view the operative field. Both of these limitations were rectified with the incorporation of the videolaparoscope.[62,63] These advances made it possible to treat even the most extensive pathology laparoscopy.[64–66]

Large case-control series were conducted in 2005 through 2008 confirming the comparable efficacy of open and laparoscopic approaches to ovarian cancer staging. Childers and coworkers suggested that laparoscopy may offer an advantage in the management of early ovarian cancer by allowing better visualization of the subdiaphragmatic areas, the obturator spaces, the anterior and posterior cul-de-sacs, as well as magnification and consequent detection of smaller lesions that may be missed on laparotomy.[67] One of the first implementations of laparoscopy was reported by Bagley and colleagues, who described visualization of diaphragmatic metastases that had been missed at the time of laparotomy.[68] The safety of a laparoscopic approach is also suggested in several studies with outcomes rivaling those reported in the literature for laparotomy. Nezhat and coworkers reported laparoscopic treatment and staging of early ovarian cancer in a case series of 36 patients with the longest recorded mean follow-up to date.[69] The mean number of peritoneal biopsies, paraaortic nodes, and pelvic nodes were 6, 12.2, and 14.8, respectively. The mean duration of follow-up was 55.9 months, and there was a demonstrated 100% overall survival rate with no recurrence.

Advanced stage invasive and recurrent ovarian cancer

A majority of patients with epithelial ovarian cancer are diagnosed with either International Federation of Gynecology and Obstetrics (FIGO) stage III or IV disease. The mainstay of treatment includes optimal surgical cytoreduction followed by platinum-based combination chemotherapy. Clinical risk factors that contribute to poor prognosis include FIGO stage IV disease, residual tumor, greater than 20 residual lesions, more than 1 L of ascites, poor performance status, older age, poor histology, high tumor grade, and high postoperative CA-125 levels. Complete surgical staging and/or debulking includes total abdominal hysterectomy, bilateral salpingo-oophorectomy, omentectomy, pelvic and paraoartic lymphadencectomy, and radical resection of all visible disease. In some cases, resecting portions of the small bowel

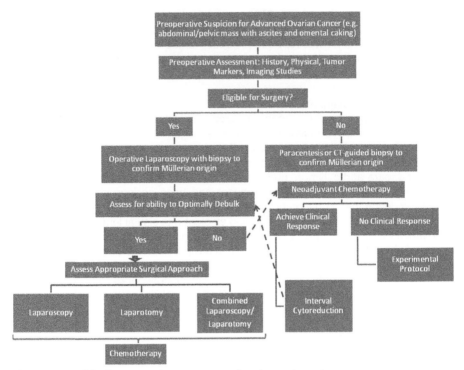

Fig. 2. Protocol for laparoscopic management in advanced ovarian cancer.

or colon may be necessary; therefore, preoperative bowel preparation may be warranted, as is a discussion during the informed consent process about possible bowel resection and diverting colostomy.

Laparoscopy can be used to effectively treat ovarian, primary peritoneal, and fallopian tube malignancies. As the use of laparoscopy has increased in gynecologic oncology, several applications have emerged in the literature: as a triage tool for resectability, as a method for second look evaluation and as a mode to select cases for primary or recurrent cytoreduction.[5] An algorithm, such as the one illustrated in **Fig. 2**, is useful in the management of presumed advanced ovarian cancer given modern technology and appropriate surgical ability. A patient can be optimally debulked to no macrosomic disease, as several studies have demonstrated.[70–72] Laparoscopy can be an ideal mode to assess the patient for suitability for cytoreduction as well. If the patient cannot be debulked, she can receive neoadjuvant chemotherapy. Receiving initial chemotherapy does not necessarily compromise the survival rate, as shown in a recent study by Vergote and colleagues.[73] In fact, chemotherapy can lead to significant tumor reduction making the patient a candidate for successful interval cytoreduction. The patient can then undergo cytoreductive surgery laparoscopically or via laparotomy depending on her unique situation.

Amara and colleagues first reported a small case series that included complete laparoscopic management of advanced or recurrent ovarian cancer.[70] All patients did well postoperatively. One patient died due to recurrent disease after declining further intervention. Nezhat and coworkers published a case series of 32 patients with advanced ovarian cancer and demonstrated that a complete debulking procedure can be performed laparoscopically in advanced cases.[71] Seventeen patients underwent laparoscopic procedures, while 11 patients underwent laparotomy. The estimated blood loss and hospital stay were not different between the 2 groups. The median time to recurrence was 31.7 months in the laparoscopy group and 21.5 months in the laparotomy group. These data illustrate that laparoscopy is a technically feasible approach in surgical management in selected patients with advanced ovarian malignancy without compromising survival.

Recent publications have explored the role of robotic procedures in the management of ovarian malignancy. Magrina and colleagues looked at perioperative and survival results in woman with ovarian cancer who underwent laparoscopic, robotic, and laparotomy procedures for management of their malignancy. They concluded that the laparoscopic and robotic approaches were preferred in patients requiring primary tumor excision alone or in addition to one additional major procedure. By contrast, laparotomy was preferred in patients with major disease requiring 2 or more additional procedures. Survival was not affected by the approach.[72]

SUMMARY

With the continued expansion of endoscopic techniques and instruments, laparoscopy and minimally invasive techniques are quickly emerging as a feasible alternative to laparotomy in managing adnexal masses and ovarian cancer. Laparoscopy has the potential to completely and successfully treat both benign and malignant adnexal pathology while decreasing unnecessary morbidity among patients. Further advances in technology, techniques, and instruments can only increase this potential.

REFERENCES

1. ACOG Practice Bulletin. Management of adnexal masses. Obstet Gynecol 2007;110: 201–14.
2. Givens V, Mitchell GE, Harraway-Smith C, et al. Diagnosis and management of adnexal masses. Am Fam Physician 2009;80:815–20.
3. Clarke-Pearson DL. Clinical practice. Screening for ovarian cancer. N Engl J Med 2009;361:170-17.
4. Schwartz PE. Nongenetic screening of ovarian malignancies. Obstet Gynecol Clin North Am 2001;28:637–51, vii.
5. Liu CS, Nagarsheth NP, Nezhat FR. Laparoscopy and ovarian cancer: a paradigm change in the management of ovarian cancer? J Minim Invasive Gynecol 2009;16: 250–62.
6. Hoffman MS. Overview of the evaluation and management of adnexal masses. UpToDate, September 29, 2010.
7. Russell DJ. The female pelvic mass. Diagnosis and management. Med Clin North Am 1995;79:1481–93.
8. Goff BA, Mandel LS, Melancon CH, et al. Frequency of symptoms of ovarian cancer in women presenting to primary care clinics. JAMA 2004;291:2705–12.
9. Cannistra SA. Cancer of the ovary. N Engl J Med 2004;351:2519–29.
10. Hennessy BT, Coleman RL, Markman M. Ovarian cancer. Lancet 2009;374: 1371–82.
11. Morch LS, Lokkegaard E, Andreasen AH, et al. Hormone therapy and ovarian cancer. JAMA 2009;302:298–305.
12. Beral V, Bull D, Green J, et al. Ovarian cancer and hormone replacement therapy in the Million Women Study. Lancet 2007;369:1703–10.

13. Rodriguez C, Patel AV, Calle EE, et al. Estrogen replacement therapy and ovarian cancer mortality in a large prospective study of US women. JAMA 2001;285: 1460–5.
14. Pados G, Tsolakidis D, Bontis J. Laparoscopic management of the adnexal mass. Ann N Y Acad Sci 2006;1092:211–28.
15. Parker WH, Berek JS. Laparoscopic management of the adnexal mass. Obstet Gynecol Clin North Am 1994;21:79–92.
16. Nezhat F, Datta MS, Hanson V, et al. The relationship of endometriosis and ovarian malignancy: a review. Fertil Steril 2008;90:1559–70.
17. Boyd J, Sonoda Y, Federici MG, et al. Clinicopathologic features of BRCA-linked and sporadic ovarian cancer. JAMA 2000;283:2260–5.
18. Agency for Healthcare Research and Quality. Management of adnexal mass. Evidence Based Report/Technology Assessment No. 130. AHRQ. Rockville, MD: Author.
19. Padilla LA, Radosevich DM, Milad MP. Limitations of the pelvic examination for evaluation of the female pelvic organs. Int J Gynaecol Obstet 2005;88:84–8.
20. Crayford TJ, Campbell S, Bourne TH, et al. Benign ovarian cysts and ovarian cancer: a cohort study with implications for screening. Lancet 2000;355:1060–3.
21. McDonald JM, Doran S, DeSimone CP, et al. Predicting risk of malignancy in adnexal masses. Obstet Gynecol 2010;115:687–94.
22. Pavlik EJ, Saunders BA, Doran S, et al. The search for meaning: symptoms and transvaginal sonography screening for ovarian cancer: predicting malignancy. Cancer 2009;115:3689–98.
23. Rossi A, Braghin C, Soldano F, et al. A proposal for a new scoring system to evaluate pelvic masses: Pelvic Masses Score (PMS). Eur J Obstet Gynecol Reprod Biol 2011.
24. van den Akker PA, Aalders AL, Snijders MP, et al. Evaluation of the Risk of Malignancy Index in daily clinical management of adnexal masses. Gynecol Oncol 2010;116: 384–8.
25. Clarke SE, Grimshaw R, Rittenberg P, et al. Risk of malignancy index in the evaluation of patients with adnexal masses. J Obstet Gynaecol Can 2009;31:440–5.
26. Guerriero S, Mais V, Ajossa S, et al. The role of endovaginal ultrasound in differentiating endometriomas from other ovarian cysts. Clin Exp Obstet Gynecol 1995;22:20–2.
27. Kupfer MC, Schwimer SR, Lebovic J. Transvaginal sonographic appearance of endometriomata: spectrum of findings. J Ultrasound Med 1992;11:129–33.
28. Ekici E, Soysal M, Kara S, et al. The efficiency of ultrasonography in the diagnosis of dermoid cysts. Zentralbl Gynakol 1996;118:136–41.
29. Guerriero S, Ajossa S, Lai MP, et al. Transvaginal ultrasonography associated with colour Doppler energy in the diagnosis of hydrosalpinx. Hum Reprod 2000;15:1568–72.
30. Bharwani N, Reznek RH, Rockall AG. Ovarian cancer management: the role of imaging and diagnostic challenges. Eur J Radiol 2011;78:41–51.
31. Screening for ovarian cancer: recommendation statement. Ann Fam Med 2004;2: 260–2.
32. NIH Consensus Conference. Ovarian cancer. Screening, treatment, and follow-up. NIH Consensus Development Panel on Ovarian Cancer. JAMA 1995;273:491–7.
33. van Nagell JR Jr, DePriest PD, Reedy MB, et al. The efficacy of transvaginal sonographic screening in asymptomatic women at risk for ovarian cancer. Gynecol Oncol 2000;77:350–6.
34. Menon U, Gentry-Maharaj A, Hallett R, et al. Sensitivity and specificity of multimodal and ultrasound screening for ovarian cancer, and stage distribution of detected cancers: results of the prevalence screen of the UK Collaborative Trial of Ovarian Cancer Screening (UKCTOCS). Lancet Oncol 2009;10:327–40.

35. Buys SS, Partridge E, Greene MH, et al. Ovarian cancer screening in the Prostate, Lung, Colorectal and Ovarian (PLCO) cancer screening trial: findings from the initial screen of a randomized trial. Am J Obstet Gynecol 2005;193:1630–9.
36. Das PM, Bast RC Jr. Early detection of ovarian cancer. Biomark Med 2008;2:291–303.
37. Helzlsouer KJ, Bush TL, Alberg AJ, et al. Prospective study of serum CA-125 levels as markers of ovarian cancer. JAMA 1993;269:1123–6.
38. Malkasian GD Jr, Knapp RC, Lavin PT, et al. Preoperative evaluation of serum CA 125 levels in premenopausal and postmenopausal patients with pelvic masses: discrimination of benign from malignant disease. Am J Obstet Gynecol 1988;159:341–6.
39. Nolen B, Velikokhatnaya L, Marrangoni A, et al. Serum biomarker panels for the discrimination of benign from malignant cases in patients with an adnexal mass. Gynecol Oncol 2010;117:440–5.
40. Jacob F, Meier M, Caduff R, et al. No benefit from combining HE4 and CA125 as ovarian tumor markers in a clinical setting. Gynecol Oncol 2011.
41. Greenlee RT, Kessel B, Williams CR, et al. Prevalence, incidence, and natural history of simple ovarian cysts among women >55 years old in a large cancer screening trial. Am J Obstet Gynecol 2010;202:373, e1–9.
42. ACOG Practice Bulletin No. 110: noncontraceptive uses of hormonal contraceptives. Obstet Gynecol 2010;115:206–18.
43. ACOG Committee Opinion: number 280, December 2002. The role of the generalist obstetrician-gynecologist in the early detection of ovarian cancer. Obstet Gynecol 2002;100:1413–6.
44. Nezhat F, Nezhat C, Welander CE, et al. Four ovarian cancers diagnosed during laparoscopic management of 1011 women with adnexal masses. Am J Obstet Gynecol 1992;167:790–6.
45. Mahdavi A, Berker B, Nezhat C, et al. Laparoscopic management of ovarian cysts. Obstet Gynecol Clin North Am 2004;31:581–92, ix.
46. Nezhat C, Winer WK, Nezhat F. Laparoscopic removal of dermoid cysts. Obstet Gynecol 1989;73:278–81.
47. Nezhat CR, Kalyoncu S, Nezhat CH, et al. Laparoscopic management of ovarian dermoid cysts: ten years' experience. JSLS 1999;3:179–84.
48. Serafini P, Kerin J, Marrs R. Management of unexpected ovarian dermoid cyst during laparoscopy for oocyte pickup. Fertil Steril 1987;48:146–8.
49. Hakim-Elahi E. Laparoscopic removal of dermoid cysts. Obstet Gynecol 1989;74:140.
50. Nezhat F, Nezhat C. Operative laparoscopy for the treatment of ovarian remnant syndrome. Fertil Steril 1992;57:1003–7.
51. Mahdavi A, Berker B, Nezhat C, et al. Laparoscopic management of ovarian remnant. Obstet Gynecol Clin North Am 2004;31:593–7, ix.
52. Allen DG. The retained ovary and the residual ovary syndrome. Aust N Z J Obstet Gynaecol 1998;38:446–7.
53. Koch MO, Coussens D, Burnett L. The ovarian remnant syndrome and ureteral obstruction: medical management. J Urol 1994;152:158–60.
54. Kho RM, Magrina JF, Magtibay PM. Pathologic findings and outcomes of a minimally invasive approach to ovarian remnant syndrome. Fertil Steril 2007;87:1005–9.
55. Abu-Rafeh B, Vilos GA, Misra M. Frequency and laparoscopic management of ovarian remnant syndrome. J Am Assoc Gynecol Laparosc 2003;10:33–7.
56. El-Minawi AM, Howard FM. Operative laparoscopic treatment of ovarian retention syndrome. J Am Assoc Gynecol Laparosc 1999;6:297–302.

57. Cadron I, Leunen K, Van Gorp T, et al. Management of borderline ovarian neoplasms. J Clin Oncol 2007;25:2928–37.
58. Nezhat C, Nezhat F, Burrell M. Laparoscopically-assisted hysterectomy for the management of a borderline ovarian tumor: a case report. J Laparoendosc Surg 1992;2:167–9.
59. Iglesias DA, Ramirez PT. Role of minimally invasive surgery in staging of ovarian cancer. Curr Treat Options Oncol 2011.
60. Nezhat C, Crowgey SR, Garrison CP. Surgical treatment of endometriosis via laser laparoscopy. Fertil Steril 1986;45:778–83.
61. Nezhat C, Nezhat C, Nezhat F, editors. Nezhat's operative gynecologic laparoscopy and hysteroscopy. New York (NY): Cambridge University Press; 2008.
62. Kelley WE Jr. The evolution of laparoscopy and the revolution in surgery in the decade of the 1990s. JSLS 2008;12:351–7.
63. Pappas TN, Jacobs DO. Laparoscopic resection for colon cancer–the end of the beginning? N Engl J Med 2004;350:2091–2.
64. Nezhat CN, Nezhat F, Silfen SL. Laparoscopic hysterectomy and bilateral salpingo-oophorectomy using multifire GIA surgical stapler. J Gynecol Surg 1990;6:185.
65. Nezhat CR, Burrell MO, Nezhat FR, et al. Laparoscopic radical hysterectomy with paraaortic and pelvic node dissection. Am J Obstet Gynecol 1992;166:864–5.
66. Amara DP, Nezhat C, Teng NN, et al. Operative laparoscopy in the management of ovarian cancer. Surg Laparosc Endosc 1996;6:38–45.
67. Childers JM, Lang J, Surwit EA, et al. Laparoscopic surgical staging of ovarian cancer. Gynecol Oncol 1995;59:25–33.
68. Bagley CM Jr, Young RC, Schein PS, et al. Ovarian carcinoma metastatic to the diaphragm—frequently undiagnosed at laparotomy. A preliminary report. Am J Obstet Gynecol 1973;116:397–400.
69. Nezhat FR, Ezzati M, Chuang L, et al. Laparoscopic management of early ovarian and fallopian tube cancers: surgical and survival outcome. Am J Obstet Gynecol 2009; 200:83 e1–6.
70. Amara DP, Nezhat C, Teng NN, et al. Operative laparoscopy in the management of ovarian cancer. Surg Laparosc Endosc 1996;6:38–45.
71. Nezhat FR, DeNoble SM, Liu CS, et al. The safety and efficacy of laparoscopic surgical staging and debulking of apparent advanced stage ovarian, fallopian tube, and primary peritoneal cancers. JSLS 2010;14:155–68.
72. Magrina JF, Zanagnolo V, Noble BN, et al. Robotic approach for ovarian cancer: perioperative and survival results and comparison with laparoscopy and laparotomy. Gynecol Oncol 2011;121:100–5.
73. Vergote I, Trope CG, Amant F, et al. Neoadjuvant chemotherapy or primary surgery in stage IIIC or IV ovarian cancer. N Engl J Med 2010;363:943–53.

Surgical Treatment of Endometriosis

Fred M. Howard, MS, MD[a,b],*

KEYWORDS

- Pelvic pain • Endometriosis • Laparoscopy
- Dysmenorrhea

Endometriosis is the presence of tissue with the histologic appearance of endometrium outside of the endometrial cavity. Its prevalence is not known, but it is estimated to affect 10% to 15% of women of reproductive age.[1] It is an enigmatic disease in that it may cause no symptoms in some women, yet result in incapacitating pain or resistant infertility in others. It may behave in a manner similar to malignancy in many women, with widespread and even metastatic disease, but differs from a malignancy in that it is almost never a source of mortality.

When endometriosis is symptomatic, it classically presents with pelvic pain, an adnexal mass, or infertility. The most common pelvic pain symptom is dysmenorrhea, occurring in more than 90% of women with endometriosis associated pelvic pain.[2] Dyspareunia and non-menstrual chronic pelvic pain are also common, occurring in 40% to 60% of symptomatic women. The physical examination is often normal, even in women with significant pelvic pain symptoms. Findings on examination suggestive of endometriosis include focal areas of pelvic tenderness, uterosacral ligament tenderness or nodularity, an adnexal mass, a fixed tender retroverted uterus, significant cervical deviation, significant vaginal allodynia, and significant cul-de-sac tenderness or nodularity. Published clinical evidence suggests that the positive predictive value of a clinical diagnosis of endometriosis is about 80%.[3] Unpublished data from our center suggest that the positive predictive value of a clinical diagnosis is about 65% and the negative predictive value is about 75%. The accuracy of clinical diagnosis is sufficient that most experts agree that empiric medical treatment without histologic confirmation is appropriate for many women with symptoms suggestive of endometriosis. However, actual

Disclosure: The author serves as a consultant for Ethicon Womens Health and Urology, a speaker for Abbott Laboratories, and a speaker for Ortho Womens Health and Urology.

[a] Department of Obstetrics and Gynecology, University of Rochester School of Medicine and Dentistry, 601 Elmwood Avenue, Box 668, Rochester, NY 14642, USA

[b] International Pelvic Pain Society, Two Woodfield Lake, 1100 East Woodfield Road, Suite 520, Schaumburg, IL 60173, USA

* Corresponding author. Department of Obstetrics and Gynecology, University of Rochester School of Medicine and Dentistry, 601 Elmwood Avenue, Box 668, Rochester, NY 14642, USA.

E-mail address: fred_howard@urmc.rochester.edu

Obstet Gynecol Clin N Am 38 (2011) 677–686

doi:10.1016/j.ogc.2011.09.004

0889-8545/11/$ – see front matter © 2011 Elsevier Inc. All rights reserved.

obgyn.theclinics.com

diagnosis requires histologic confirmation, which is almost always obtained by laparoscopically directed biopsies.

In modern gynecologic practice, when the decision is made to perform a laparoscopy to confirm the diagnosis, the surgeon should be prepared to treat the disease surgically at the same time.[4] In almost all cases, several types of medical treatment should have been used already without adequate pain relief, or the laparoscopy is for treatment of infertility. In both circumstances, optimal results require surgical debulking of endometriotic lesions, if present. In this review, only principles for optimal treatment of pelvic pain are discussed, not treatment of infertility.

PITFALLS IN SURGICAL MANAGEMENT

There are at least 3 major pitfalls related to surgical treatment of endometriosis-associated pelvic pain.

There is Not a Direct Cause and Effect Relationship of Endometriosis and Pelvic Pain in All Women

All gynecologists know that endometriosis is not always symptomatic and that many women with endometriosis do not have significant pelvic pain. Yet, when a woman has pelvic pain and is then found to have endometriosis, it is automatically assumed that the endometriosis is the cause of pain. In fact, asymptomatic endometriosis is probably just as likely in women with pelvic pain as it is in women without pelvic pain.

There are many other diagnoses that are at least as common pain generators as endometriosis in women with chronic pelvic pain, in particular, irritable bowel syndrome, interstitial cystitis/painful bladder syndrome, and myofascial pain syndrome. It is important that the history and physical examination be consistent with endometriosis-associated pelvic pain, and that other diagnoses be eliminated, before pain is exclusively attributed to endometriosis. For example, in our pelvic pain center only 18% of women with endometriosis have only endometriosis as a pain-related diagnosis: 31% also have irritable bowel syndrome, 32% also have interstitial cystitis/painful bladder syndrome, 18% also have provoked vestibulodynia, and 21% also have myofascial pain syndrome of the abdomen or pelvic floor.[5] Although it is crucial that all possible pain generators be treated, it is usually not possible to discern the degree of pain that may attributed to each, and this is true for endometriosis as well. It serves the woman with chronic pelvic pain poorly if she is diagnosed with endometriosis based on laparoscopic findings and no other potential etiologies are sought, even though the history is not consistent with endometriosis or the response to treatment for endometriosis is poor. Again, it is important to consider that the laparoscopic finding of endometriosis may be incidental and nonsymptomatic, or it may be symptomatic but represent only one of several important pain-related diagnoses.

Patients with Pelvic Pain may be Misdiagnosed with Endometriosis

As alluded to, endometriosis is not a clinical diagnosis but rather is a histologic diagnosis. The clinical diagnosis of endometriosis has a positive predictive value of 65% to 80% and a negative predictive value of about 75%. Although these values are high enough to justify empiric treatment, they are not sufficient to base the diagnosis solely on clinical characteristics.

Additionally, endometriosis is not a visual diagnosis. Many gynecologic surgeons have been comfortable with solely a visual diagnosis of endometriosis based on the appearance of lesions at the time of laparoscopy. Published evidence shows that this opinion is flawed, and in fact that a visual diagnosis of endometriosis at the time of

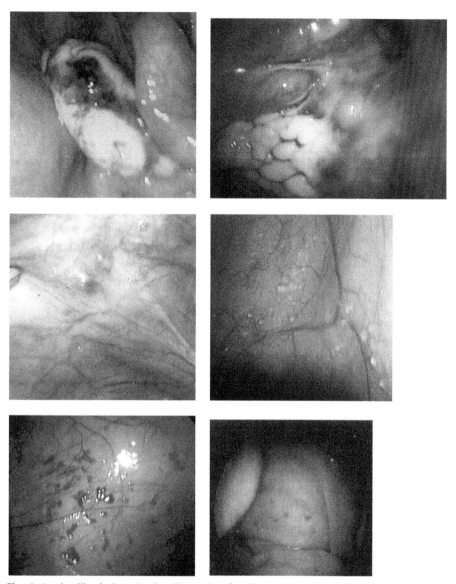

Fig. 1. Look alike lesions in the diagnosis of endometriosis. The lesions on the left are endometriosis and those on the right are not.

laparoscopy is probably even less accurate than a clinical diagnosis without laparoscopy. The best data on this issue suggest that a visual diagnosis of endometriosis has only a 45% positive predictive value.[6] This is really not surprising when one considers the variety of appearances that endometriosis can manifest (**Fig. 1**).

Data from conscious laparoscopic pain mapping suggest that histologic confirmation is very relevant in the evaluation of chronic pelvic pain. In a series of 50 patients successfully laparoscopically pain mapped, 15 had visual findings that were consistent with the diagnosis of endometriosis.[7] Only 7 of these patients had reproduction of their pelvic pain upon stimulation of these lesions and all 7 of these patients had histologic confirmation of the diagnosis of endometriosis. In contrast, in the 8 patients whose lesions did not reproduce their pain, only 2 had a histologic diagnosis of endometriosis. In other words, 7 (78%) of 9 patients with endometriosis had pain produced with stimulation of the lesions, whereas 0 of 6 patients had pain produced with stimulation of lesions that were visually thought to be endometriosis but were not ($P = .007$). This clearly points out the error in attributing pelvic pain to endometriosis without a histologic confirmation of the diagnosis.

Endometriosis may be Inadequately Treated at the Time of Surgery

There are 2 major reasons for inadequate operative treatment. One is the lack of sufficient surgical skills to be able to remove all endometriotic lesions. The other is the failure to remove all lesions that may possibly be endometriosis lesions.

A discussion of the surgical skills that should be mandatory before undertaking laparoscopic evaluation for endometriosis is fraught with controversy. It is beyond the scope of this review to debate the political, economic, and social implications of requiring that any surgeon who operates on a woman with pelvic pain, with the anticipation of a diagnosis of endometriosis, must have the requisite skills to appropriately debulk and destroy the disease, regardless of its severity. Some experts have suggested that endometriosis patients should only receive care at centers of excellence dedicated to the management of endometriosis.[8] Such recommendations probably deserve consideration and study.

The second reason for inadequate surgery—the failure to recognize and remove all endometriosis lesions—is the converse side of the discussion of inaccurate diagnosis based on visual findings. Just as the diagnosis can be wrong because of the variety of possible appearances of endometriosis, the treatment can be incomplete unless all lesions that have an appearance that could possibly be endometriosis are removed or destroyed. Thus, not just classic powder burn lesions or endometriomas must be removed, but also clear vesicular lesions, red lesions, brown lesions, peritoneal pockets, glandular-appearing lesions, and so on. Our preference is to excise almost all lesions for histologic evaluation so that a sense of the magnitude or load of disease can be assessed, based on the number of actual endometriosis lesions. It is well known that classic staging is not particularly helpful the patient with pelvic pain.

Of course, this means that all potential locations of endometriosis in the pelvis and abdomen must be evaluated, with special attention to the most common sites: The posterior cul de sac, uterosacral ligaments, ovaries, ovarian fossae, anterior cul de sac, appendix, and ileocecal area. There are a few published suggestions to improve visualization that, although not well studied, seem to be clinically useful. "Near-contact" laparoscopy allows about an 8-fold magnification so that even very small lesions can be seen. Of course, this requires patience to thoroughly evaluate the entire pelvic with this technique. "Blood painting," which means using blood to paint the cul de sac and sidewalls of the pelvis, highlights surface irregularities that are sometimes areas of diffuse endometriosis. "Underwater examination" can be used in the cul de sac to magnify lesions to facilitate identification. Finally, preoperative imaging with ultrasonography or magnetic resonance imaging can be useful to identify occult endometriomas or invasive bladder, rectovaginal, or colorectal lesions.

SURGICAL TECHNIQUES
Laparoscopy Versus Laparotomy

There is level 1 evidence only for laparoscopic treatment of endometriosis, not laparotomic. Two randomized clinical trials of laparoscopic surgical treatment have been published. The first was a study of laser ablation of endometriosis at stages I through III.[9] At 6 months postoperatively, this study showed 62% of treated patients had decreased pain compared with 23% in the "placebo" group (number needed to treat = 2.5). It should be noted that only patients with stages II and III showed significant improvements over the control group, not patients with stage I disease. The second study was of excision of endometriosis in patients with stages II through IV disease.[10] At 6 months postoperatively, 80% of the surgically treated group reported improvement compared with only 32% in the control group (number needed to treat = 2.1). It is important to point out that in neither of these studies did conservative surgical treatment achieve 100% effectiveness and that average pain levels were decreased by approximately 50%.

Of course, full surgical debulking of endometriosis can be extremely difficult and even expert groups report the need to convert to laparotomy in 2% to 5% of cases.[11] However, in general, when laparoscopy can be done it is considered the optimal operative approach, not laparotomy, owing to decreased cost, decreased pain, decreased wound complications, and faster recovery.

Excision Versus Ablation Versus Coagulation

The technical objectives of surgery for endometriosis are to restore normal pelvic anatomy and destroy or remove all endometriosis implants. The clinical objective is to relieve pelvic pain when present, and with conservative surgery to restore or maintain fertility.[4] Although surgeons are often passionate in their arguments over the best techniques to obtain these objectives, with the exception of treatment of endometriomas, there are no data that any technique is superior. At least 2 randomized trials have evaluated excision versus ablation and neither was able to show any difference in relief of pelvic pain between the 2 techniques.[12,13] Coagulation techniques with bipolar energy have not been as well studied. One caveat regarding coagulation with bipolar forceps is that the depth of penetration of destructive energy tends to be only 2 mm; therefore, this technique is best for superficial disease. However, the expert gynecologic surgeon knows that it is important to be able to skillfully use all 3 techniques for the treatment of endometriosis. For example, a peritoneal lesion that is very small and is clearly superficial may be best treated with bipolar coagulation to minimize tissue destruction. In contrast, a deeply invasive lesion requires use of either excision or ablation. And if there is any lesion in close proximity to the ureter or on the intestine, excision without the use of thermal energy is usually most appropriate (**Fig. 2**).

In contrast, for endometriomas there are at least 4 studies that taken together show that recurrence of endometriomas is less likely with excision than with ablation or coagulation.[14–17] Additionally, there is evidence that the use of thermal energy to remove an endometrioma or to obtain hemostasis is relatively contraindicated owing to the destruction of normal ovarian tissue with resultant loss of ovarian reserve.[18]

Laparoscopic Uterine Nerve Ablation

Based on a small, randomized trial of laparoscopic uterine nerve ablation (LUNA) for the treatment of primary dysmenorrhea, published in 1987, this procedure worked its way into the armamentarium of gynecologic surgeons for the treatment of pelvic pain.[19] At 1 point, it was considered to be a routine part of the surgical treatment of women with endometriosis-associated pelvic pain.[9]

However, there are now 4 randomized, clinical trials that quite clearly show that LUNA has no role in the treatment of pelvic pain or of endometriosis-associated pelvic pain.[20–23] For endometriosis treatment, LUNA does not improve dysmenorrhea,

A   B

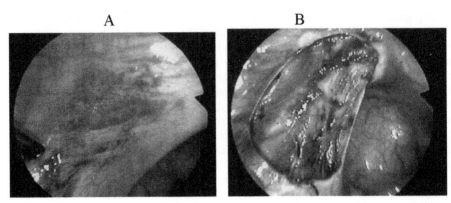

Fig. 2. Excision of peritoneal endometriosis lateral to the left uterosacral ligament and very near the left ureter. *(A)* Area of red endometriosis lesions. *(B)* As seen after excision that avoided the underlying ureter and allowed complete removal of the endometriosis .

dyspareunia, or non-menstrual pelvic pain. LUNA should not be performed for endometriosis-associated pelvic pain.

Presacral Neurectomy

There are 3 published, randomized, clinical trials that purport to study the efficacy of presacral neurectomy for the treatment of endometriosis associated pelvic pain. The first actually only randomized 8 patients because the institutional research board terminated the study based on observational data that showed efficacy.[24] The second study showed only an 8% difference between the presacral neurectomy group and group that only had endometriosis treatment.[25] The third study showed a significant improvement with the addition of presacral neurectomy to the operative treatment of endometriosis-associated pelvic pain, with a number needed to treat of 3.6 for dysmenorrhea.[26,27] However, the average decrease of visual analog scale pain scores for dysmenorrhea was only about 8 on a 100-point scale. Complications occurred in about 9% of patients, including intractable constipation in 2%. Combining the results of the last 2 studies gives an odds ratio for efficacy of presacral neurectomy for the treatment of endometriosis-associated dysmenorrhea of 3.1 (95% confidence interval, 1.6–6.2) and a number needed to treat of 4.5. Thus, although there is experimental evidence for the efficacy of including presacral neurectomy as a component of the surgical treatment of endometriosis-associated pelvic pain, the actual magnitude of pain relief, as well as the risk of bladder and bowel dysfunction, mandates that the gynecologic surgeon must carefully weigh all of these factors before the decision to perform a presacral neurectomy for endometriosis.

Preoperative Medical Treatment

Although the issue of whether to treat endometriosis preoperatively seems important, there is limited published evidence regarding the role of preoperative medical treatment for endometriosis-associated pelvic pain. One published, randomized, controlled study suggests that preoperative treatment with a gonadotropin releasing agonist for 6 months decreases the difficulty of the surgical procedure and facilitates complete debulking of endometriosis.[28] Clearly, more data would be helpful to guide the decision of whether to treat patients medically before surgical treatment.

Postoperative Medical Treatment

There are prospective, randomized control trials of postoperative treatment with rofe-coxib (no longer available in the United States),[29] danazol,[30,31] medroxyprogesterone acetate,[32] gonadotropin-releasing hormone agonists,[33] and a levonorgestrel-releasing intrauterine device.[34] All of the medical treatments seemed to decrease pain levels more than surgery alone, but only while the medications were continued. Once the medications were discontinued, pain levels in the medically treated groups rose to the same as those in the only surgically treated groups. Thus, there is no evidence of the long-lasting effectiveness owing to postoperative medical treatment. The study of postoperative levonorgestrel releasing intrauterine device showed better pain relief for dysmenorrhea and dyspareunia, but not for nonmenstrual chronic pelvic pain, compared with surgery only. Finally, there is a nonrandomized study suggesting that combining the aromatase inhibitor letrozole with norethisterone gave better postoperative pain relief than treatment with norethisterone only.[35] In this study, pain levels increased rapidly after discontinuation of medical treatment as well.

The clinical application of this evidence suggests that patients who undergo conservative surgical treatment for endometriosis-associated pelvic pain and do not desire pregnancies immediately should be medically treated postoperatively to improve their pain levels until they are ready to attempt pregnancy.

Conservative Versus Extirpative Surgery

For this discussion, extirpative surgery means the removal of 1 or both ovaries, or the uterus, and conservative surgery means the removal only of endometriosis lesions. As a general guideline, extirpative surgery should not be performed in a woman who desires the preservation of fertility. It is still common to see an endometrioma, even in an adolescent, treated by oophorectomy. With extremely rare exception, an ovary should not be removed in the woman desirous of future pregnancy. Because of the high recurrence of endometriosis, it is not reasonable to assume that preservation of 1 ovary and removal of the other is appropriate in this situation. Extirpative surgeries should only be done when preservation of fertility is no longer important to the patient.

Unfortunately, there are no well-designed clinical trials to provide guidance on the efficacies of the various extirpative options: Total hysterectomy, supracervical hysterectomy, unilateral salpingo-oophorectomy, or bilateral salpingo-oophorectomy (BSO). Anecdotal experience and observational studies suggest that pain relief is obtained in 85% to 90% of patients after treatment of endometriosis that includes total hysterectomy and BSO. There are reported cases of recurrence of endometriosis and pelvic pain after hysterectomy–BSO, but it is not common.[36] It is also not clear whether hormonal replacement significantly increases the chance of these rare recurrences. There is some suggestion that recurrence after hysterectomy–BSO is more likely, especially if all endometriosis lesions were not removed or destroyed at the time of the hysterectomy.[37] Hysterectomy without BSO seems to have a higher rate of persistent or recurrent pain, but quality data are not available and estimates are anywhere from a 15% to a 50% chance of recurrent of persistent pain if 1 or both ovaries are retained.[38] This risk must be balanced with the known decrease of life expectancy with surgical castration.[39–42] Currently there are no clear guidelines for the decision of BSO as part of extirpative surgical treatment and each case should be individualized.

There are case reports suggesting the supracervical hysterectomy increases the likelihood of recurrent endometriosis and pain compared with total hysterectomy.[43] More data are needed before any definitive statement can be made about this decision. As with BSO, it seems most appropriate to base the decision on the needs of the individual patient at this time.

SUMMARY

In this review, the pitfalls that still exist with the surgical treatment of endometriosis-associated pelvic pain have been discussed and the best evidence regarding various aspects of surgical techniques have been reviewed. When laparoscopy is performed to evaluate a woman with pelvic pain symptoms, it is important she be counseled that the primary function of the surgery is to confirm the presence (and allow surgical treatment) of endometriosis, and that it is not the penultimate diagnostic modality for her pelvic pain. There are many etiologies of pelvic pain that present with symptoms resembling those of endometriosis-associated pelvic pain that are not diagnosable with laparoscopy, such as interstitial cystitis and irritable bowel syndrome. It is unfortunate that many women are left with the belief that if a laparoscopy fails to provide a diagnosis of a pain generator, then it means there are no diagnoses other than that the "pain is in her head," often disparagingly termed "supratentorial" by clinicians. In fact, the pain-related diagnoses that are amenable to and possibly require a laparoscopy are quite limited, a group of diagnoses that this author terms the "dirty dozen" because there are just 12, and only the first 4 have good evidence to clearly associate them with chronic pelvic pain:

1. Endometriosis
2. Ovarian remnant syndrome
3. Pelvic inflammatory disease
4. Tuberculous salpingitis
5. Adhesions
6. Benign cystic mesothelioma
7. Postoperative peritoneal cysts
8. Adnexal cysts (nonendometriotic)
9. Chronic ectopic pregnancy
10. Endosalpingiosis
11. Residual accessory ovary
12. Hernias: ventral, inguinal, femoral, spigelian.

I would argue that diagnostic laparoscopy in modern gynecology has a limited, if any, role, and that when laparoscopy is planned for women with chronic pelvic pain, it should be with a very high suspicion of a diagnosis and with plans to treat the disease operatively. In this era, a negative diagnostic laparoscopy should be a rare event.

REFERENCES

1. Gao X, Outley J, Botteman M, et al. Economic burden of endometriosis. Fertil Steril 2006;86:1561–72.
2. Ballweg ML. Impact of endometriosis on women's health: comparative historical data show that the earlier the onset, the more severe the disease. Best Pract Res Clin Obstet Gynaecol 2004;18:201–18.
3. Ling FW. Randomized controlled trial of depot leuprolide in patients with chronic pelvic pain and clinically suspected endometriosis. Pelvic Pain Study Group. Obstet Gynecol 1999;93:51–8.
4. Howard FM. Laparoscopic evaluation and treatment of women with chronic pelvic pain. J Am Assoc Gynecol Laparosc 1994;1:325–31.
5. Droz J, Howard FM. Use of the Short-Form McGill Pain Questionnaire as a diagnostic tool in women with chronic pelvic pain. J Minim Invasive Gynecol 2011;18:211–7.

6. Walter AJ, Hentz JG, Magtibay PM, et al. Endometriosis: correlation between histologic and visual findings at laparoscopy. Am J Obstet Gynecol 2001;184:1407–11.
7. Howard FM, El-Minawi AM, Sanchez RA. Conscious pain mapping by laparoscopy in women with chronic pelvic pain. Obstet Gynecol 2000;96:934–9.
8. D'Hooghe T, Hummelshoj L. Multi-disciplinary centres/networks of excellence for endometriosis management and research: a proposal. Hum Reprod 2006;21: 2743–8.
9. Sutton CJ, Ewen SP, Whitelaw N, et al. Prospective, randomized, double-blind, controlled trial of laser laparoscopy in the treatment of pelvic pain associated with minimal, mild, and moderate endometriosis. Fertil Steril 1994;62:696–700.
10. Abbott J, Hawe J, Hunter D, et al. Laparoscopic excision of endometriosis: a randomized, placebo-controlled trial. Fertil Steril 2004;82:878–84.
11. Busacca M, Marana R, Caruana P, et al. Recurrence of ovarian endometrioma after laparoscopic excision. Am J Obstet Gynecol 1999;180:519–23.
12. Healey M, Ang WC, Cheng C. Surgical treatment of endometriosis: a prospective randomized double-blinded trial comparing excision and ablation. Fertil Steril 2010; 94:2536–40.
13. Wright J, Lotfallah H, Jones K, et al. A randomized trial of excision versus ablation for mild endometriosis. Fertil Steril 2005;83:1830–6.
14. Fayez JA, Vogel MF. Comparison of different treatment methods of endometriomas by laparoscopy. Obstet Gynecol 1991;78:660–5.
15. Hemmings R, Bissonnette F, Bouzayen R. Results of laparoscopic treatments of ovarian endometriomas: laparoscopic ovarian fenestration and coagulation. Fertil Steril 1998;70:527–9.
16. Beretta P, Franchi M, Ghezzi F, et al. Randomized clinical trial of two laparoscopic treatments of endometriomas: cystectomy versus drainage and coagulation. Fertil Steril 1998;70:1176–80.
17. Saleh A, Tulandi T. Reoperation after laparoscopic treatment of ovarian endometriomas by excision and by fenestration. Fertil Steril 1999;72:322–4.
18. Busacca M, Riparini J, Somigliana E, et al. Postsurgical ovarian failure after laparoscopic excision of bilateral endometriomas. Am J Obstet Gynecol 2006;195:421–5.
19. Lichten EM, Bombard J. Surgical treatment of primary dysmenorrhea with laparoscopic uterine nerve ablation. J Reprod Med 1987;32:37–41.
20. Sutton C, Pooley AS, Jones KD, et al. A prospective, randomized, double-blind controlled trial of laparoscopic uterine nerve ablation in the treatment of pelvic pain associated with endometriosis. Gynaecol Endosc 2001;10:6.
21. Vercellini P, Aimi G, Busacca M, et al. Laparoscopic uterosacral ligament resection for dysmenorrhea associated with endometriosis: results of a randomized, controlled trial. Fertil Steril 2003;80:310–9.
22. Johnson NP, Farquhar CM, Crossley S, et al. A double-blind randomised controlled trial of laparoscopic uterine nerve ablation for women with chronic pelvic pain. BJOG 2004;111:950–9.
23. Daniels J, Gray R, Hills RK, et al. Laparoscopic uterosacral nerve ablation for alleviating chronic pelvic pain: a randomized controlled trial. JAMA 2009;302:955–61.
24. Tjaden B, Schlaff WD, Kimball A, et al. The efficacy of presacral neurectomy for the relief of midline dysmenorrhea. Obstet Gynecol 1990;76:89–91.
25. Candiani GB, Fedele L, Vercellini P, et al. Presacral neurectomy for the treatment of pelvic pain associated with endometriosis: a controlled study. Am J Obstet Gynecol 1992;167:100–3.
26. Zullo F, Palomba S, Zupi E, et al. Effectiveness of presacral neurectomy in women with severe dysmenorrhea caused by endometriosis who were treated with laparoscopic

conservative surgery: a 1-year prospective randomized double-blind controlled trial. Am J Obstet Gynecol 2003;189:5–10.

27. Zullo F, Palomba S, Zupi E, et al. Long-term effectiveness of presacral neurectomy for the treatment of severe dysmenorrhea due to endometriosis. J Am Assoc Gynecol Laparosc 2004;11:23–8.

28. Audebert A, Descamps P, Marret H, et al. Pre or post-operative medical treatment with nafarelin in stage III-IV endometriosis: a French multicenter study. Eur J Obstet Gynecol Reprod Biol 1998;79:145–8.

29. Cobellis L, Razzi S, De Simone S, et al. The treatment with a COX-2 specific inhibitor is effective in the management of pain related to endometriosis. Eur J Obstet Gynecol Reprod Biol 2004;116:100–2.

30. Bianchi S, Busacca M, Agnoli B, et al. Effects of 3 month therapy with danazol after laparoscopic surgery for stage III/IV endometriosis: a randomized study. Hum Reprod 1999;14:1335–7.

31. Morgante G, Ditto A, La Marca A, et al. Low-dose danazol after combined surgical and medical therapy reduces the incidence of pelvic pain in women with moderate and severe endometriosis. Hum Reprod 1999;14:2371–4.

32. Telimaa S, Ronnberg L, Kauppila A. Placebo-controlled comparison of danazol and high-dose medroxyprogesterone acetate in the treatment of endometriosis after conservative surgery. Gynecol Endocrinol 1987;1:363–71.

33. Hornstein MD, Hemmings R, Yuzpe AA, et al. Use of nafarelin versus placebo after reductive laparoscopic surgery for endometriosis. Fertil Steril 1997;68:860–4.

34. Vercellini P, Frontino G, De Giorgi O, et al. Comparison of a levonorgestrel-releasing intrauterine device versus expectant management after conservative surgery for symptomatic endometriosis: a pilot study. Fertil Steril 2003;80:305–9.

35. Ferrero S, Camerini G, Seracchioli R, et al. Letrozole combined with norethisterone acetate compared with norethisterone acetate alone in the treatment of pain symptoms caused by endometriosis. Hum Reprod 2009;24:3033–41.

36. Redwine DB. Endometriosis persisting after castration: clinical characteristics and results of surgical management. Obstet Gynecol 1994;83:405–13.

37. Clayton RD, Hawe JA, Love JC, et al. Recurrent pain after hysterectomy and bilateral salpingo-oophorectomy for endometriosis: evaluation of laparoscopic excision of residual endometriosis. Br J Obstet Gynaecol 1999;106:740–4.

38. Namnoum AB, Hickman TN, Goodman SB, et al. Incidence of symptom recurrence after hysterectomy for endometriosis. Fertil Steril 1995;64:898–902.

39. Parker WH. Bilateral oophorectomy versus ovarian conservation: effects on long-term women's health. J Minim Invasive Gynecol 2010;17:161–6.

40. Parker WH, Broder MS, Chang E, et al. Ovarian conservation at the time of hysterectomy and long-term health outcomes in the nurses' health study. Obstet Gynecol 2009;113:1027–37.

41. Parker WH, Broder MS, Liu Z, et al. Ovarian conservation at the time of hysterectomy for benign disease. Clin Obstet Gynecol 2007;50:354–61.

42. Parker WH, Broder MS, Liu Z, et al. Ovarian conservation at the time of hysterectomy for benign disease. Obstet Gynecol 2005;106:219–26.

43. Nezhat CH, Nezhat F, Roemisch M, et al. Laparoscopic trachelectomy for persistent pelvic pain and endometriosis after supracervical hysterectomy. Fertil Steril 1996;66: 925–8.

Electrosurgery: Principles and Practice to Reduce Risk and Maximize Efficacy

Andrew I. Brill, MD

KEYWORDS
- Blend • Coag • Cut • Electrosurgery
- Bipolar • Monopolar

FUNDAMENTALS OF ELECTRICITY

Electricity is a form of electromagnetic energy that flows between atoms. Electrical current (I) is defined as the amount of electricity moving through a conductor over a specific amount of time. Given a significant difference in electrical potential, electrons are set in motion in a particular direction within a conductor to carry an electrical current that is measured in amperes (A) and represents the rate of flow of electrical charge. The electromotive force that drives the current through the conductor is referred to as voltage (V). Resistance (termed impedance with high-frequency AC), is measured in Ohms and represents the property of a conductor that opposes the flow of the current (**Fig. 1**).

Electricity is governed by Ohm's Law:

$$V \text{ (voltage)} = I \text{ (current)} \times R \text{ (resistance or impedance)}$$

Current (I) is directly proportional to voltage (V) and inversely proportional to resistance (R). Greater resistance therefore requires greater voltage. If the resistance (impedance) is a fixed variable, greater voltage will create greater current. On the other hand, power (the number keyed on the electrosurgical generator [ESU]) quantifies the rate of work being done and is expressed in watts (W). Power (W) is expressed by the equation:

$$W = I \times V, \text{ or alternatively as } W = I^2 \times R \text{ and } W = V^2/R$$

When an electrode is applied to tissue with higher impedance (eg, fat), a conventional electrosurgical generator correspondingly outputs greater voltage (V) providing the power setting (W) remains unchanged. Because voltage (V) is the force that drives charged particles across a potential difference, greater voltage has the propensity to

The author has nothing to disclose.
California Pacific Medical Center, 3700 California Street, G330, San Francisco, CA 94118, USA
E-mail address: endoandy@comcast.net

Obstet Gynecol Clin N Am 38 (2011) 687–702
doi:10.1016/j.ogc.2011.09.005
0889-8545/11/$ – see front matter © 2011 Elsevier Inc. All rights reserved.

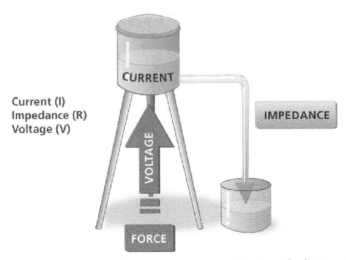

Current (I)
Impedance (R)
Voltage (V)

Fig. 1. The fundamental elements of electricity—current, resistance, and voltage—are depicted by a water tower. Just as it takes pressure to fill the reservoir, voltage is the electromotive force that drives current across an electrical circuit. As more fluid or a smaller diameter outlet would require greater pressure, greater current or increasing resistance requires higher voltage. (Ohm's law: $V = I \times R$). (*From* Brill AI. Electrosurgery: principles and practices. APGO Educational Series on Women's Health Issues. Association of Professors of Gynecology and Obstetrics; with permission. Available at: http://www.apgo.org/electrosurgery/index.html.)

produce greater lateral and deeper thermal necrosis. A "pathway" or completed circuit must exist for electrons to flow. Because energy can neither be created nor destroyed, heat is produced as the moving electrons encounter any kind of resistance—so-called resistive heating. This ability of electricity to produce work in the form of heat in living tissue is central to the mechanism of electrosurgery. The surgeon's goal during the use of electrosurgery is to attain anatomic dissection with hemostasis while causing the least amount of collateral damage and subsequent scar tissue formation.[1]

Two types of electrical current exist: Direct current (DC) and alternating current (AC). With DC, the electrons flow in only 1 direction. With AC, the electrons constantly change direction, moving between positive and negative poles, as the current flows along a circuit The frequency at which AC oscillates between the positive and negative poles is measured in Hertz (Hz), or cycles per second (1 Hz = 1 cycle/sec). Accidental contact with household outlet current, which oscillates at 60 cycles per second (60 Hz), causes tetanic skeletal muscle contraction by depolarization of the neuromuscular junction—the so-called Faradic effects. Contact with current above 100,000 cycles per second does not cause tetany or have the potential to electrocute. Flacidity is maintained during surgery as the electrosurgical generator (ESU) converts the low frequency AC from a standard electrical outlet to very high frequency AC (300–600 kHz range). Because the frequency used for electrosurgery includes that of both radio and television signal transmission (550–880 kHz), electrosurgery current is also referred to as radiofrequency current.[2]

FUNDAMENTALS OF ELECTROSURGERY

Electrosurgery is accomplished by conducting high frequency AC through living tissue. All electrosurgical tissue effects occur from sufficiently concentrated tissue

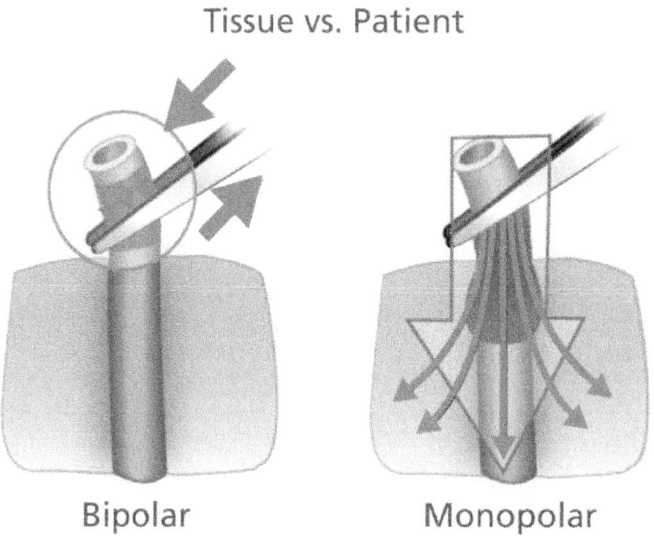

Tissue vs. Patient

Bipolar   Monopolar

Fig. 2. In bipolar electrosurgery, the current flows from the generator to the hand-held, 2-poled instrument, and back to the generator. The current does not enter the rest of the body. Tissue effects are applied only to the tissue held in the instrument. No dispersive electrode is needed. (*From* Brill Al. Electrosurgery: principles and practices. APGO Educational Series on Women's Health Issues. Association of Professors of Gynecology and Obstetrics; with permission. Available at: http://www.apgo.org/electrosurgery/index.html.)

heat, a byproduct of electrons flowing through tissue resistance. Often, the term electrocautery is erroneously used instead of electrosurgery. Electrocautery is directly burning tissue with a hot surgical instrument. On the other hand, during electrosurgery, the tissue is part of a complete electrical circuit[3] where thermal effects can be precisely moderated.

Electricity will always seek ground (the earth) by conducting along pathways of least resistance. During monopolar electrosurgery, the complete electrical circuit includes the ESU, the active and dispersive electrode, and patient's tissues.[4] Once electrical current is applied to the tissue target, it is conducted from the surgical site through a myriad of tissue pathways to a much larger surface area via the dispersive (grounding) electrode. The larger surface area and substantially lower current density prevents tissue heating sufficiently to burn. On the other hand, during bipolar electrosurgery, both electrodes are isolated to the small amount of intervening tissue at the surgical site. Thermal effects are equally distributed between the surfaces of each electrode (**Fig. 2**).

Understanding Electrosurgical Waveforms: Cut, Blend, and Coag

The AC used for electrosurgery is a sinusoidal waveform (constantly changing directions). The typical output settings labeled *cut, blend*, and *coag* on the face of conventional electrosurgical generators are simply variations of current and voltage in relation to time, called waveforms (**Fig. 3**). Despite the common presumption that the labels *cut, blend*, and *coag* are necessarily related to specific tissue effects, they are not required for any particular electrosurgical tissue endpoint.

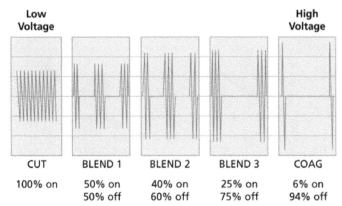

Fig. 3. Waveforms produced by ESUs range from low-voltage pure cut mode to high-voltage coagulation mode, with a variety of blend waveforms in between. (*From* Brill AI. Electrosurgery: principles and practices. APGO Educational Series on Women's Health Issues. Association of Professors of Gynecology and Obstetrics; with permission. Available at: http://www.apgo.org/electrosurgery/index.html.)

A pure *cut* waveform is an uninterrupted sine wave of low voltage. Compared with the other outputs, the average current is the highest (uninterrupted) and the peak voltage is lowest. The *blend* output should not be misconstrued as being some mixture or blend of other types of waveforms. The term *blend* refers to a blend of net surgical effects (cutting with coagulation), not a literal blend of different types of waveforms. Correctly speaking, electrosurgical generator settings in this mode (ie, *blend 1*, *blend 2*) simply produce progressive drops in average current by inserting current interruption of greater duration (ie, *blend 1* is "on" 50% of the time, *blend 2* 40%, and *blend 3* 25%). As current progressively drops with higher blend settings, the output voltage must progressively increase to conserve energy ($V = I \times R$).

The pure *coag* waveform is a highly interrupted current with frequent and prolonged gaps. Switched to this mode, significantly higher voltage is delivered, but the current is "on" (the duty cycle) only 6% of the time. Comparatively, the pure cut mode is "on" 100% of the time. To maintain the same power output (W), the significantly lower average current (I) of the coag output is automatically balanced by the generation of a higher output voltage (recall, $W = I \times V$).[1]

To achieve numerous tissue effects, the surgeon can use the electrosurgery waveforms in combination with many other factors: Power settings (W), the electrode dwell time (the length of exposure or velocity), the volume of tissue treated, the proximity of the tissue to the active electrode, and the current density. Tissue impedance (resistance), which primarily depends on water content, also affects the outcome. Impedance is high in calloused tissues, moderate in adipose tissues, and very low in vascular tissues. Moreover, impedance of tissues is dynamic during electrosurgery. For example, as tissue coagulates and water evaporates, impedance rises—at times to the point that the current is inhibited from flowing through the tissue. If the surgeon increases the power setting (W) and consequently the output voltage (V), the current (I) is more likely to seek an alternate pathway via the least resistance to the ground, which may lead to thermal injury. Therefore, it is advisable to use the lowest power setting to achieve the desired tissue effects.[4]

BIPOLAR AND MONOPOLAR ELECTROSURGERY
Bipolar Electrosurgery

Electrosurgery is traditionally described as either in bipolar or monopolar mode. In fact, all electrosurgery is intrinsically bipolar, owing to the use of AC. With the conventional bipolar mode, the patient is in essence not part of the circuit; the current does not enter the patient's body beyond the immediate surgical site (see **Fig. 2**). Rather than coursing through the body, the flow of AC is symmetrically distributed, reversing direction every half cycle, and is conducted from the generator to 1 electrode (of a 2-poled surgical instrument), through the tissue being grasped or contacted, to the second electrode, and back to the generator. In the bipolar mode, the energy is delivered and returned at the same site with no need for a large dispersive electrode.[1]

Intuitively then, bipolar electrosurgery has some advantages over monopolar electrosurgery. It is a reliable method of occluding and sealing blood vessels, and it can limit the amount of affected tissue. It also has a more limited area of thermal spread, resulting in less smoke. Because the 2 electrodes are in close proximity, it can work well under saline or nonelectrolyte solutions in the surgical field. In addition, it potentially alleviates cross-interference with implanted electrical devices such as cardiac pacemakers.[3]

Despite the isolation of tissue between the bipolar electrodes, thermal damage may occur well beyond their confines. Desiccation of tissue strongly percolates heated intracellular water into adjacent tissues. The unabated application of current can propagate a secondary thermal bloom that disruptively bubbles steam through the surrounding parenchyma. Thermal spread is best limited by terminating current on tissue whitening and when water vapor can no longer be seen to percolate from the heated tissue. Despite its propriety for determining the endpoint for bipolar tubal sterilization, use of an in-line ammeter, which meters the flow of current between the tissue and the jaws of the bipolar grasper, does not prevent this problem. Rather, it tends to promote overdesiccation of tissue. Because larger, compressed tissue pedicles can generate greater heat, unwanted thermal damage can also be minimized by selectively utilizing the sides or tips of a slightly open bipolar device to directly tamponade and then desiccate with the episodic application of current. Compared with bipolar electrosurgery, monopolar electrosurgery requires substantially higher voltage (V) to propel the current (I) along the myriad of tissue conductors between the active and dispersive electrode to complete the significantly longer electrical circuit. Although this provides a greater range of available tissue effects, it also poses increased potential for undesired effects, such as burns at the dispersive electrode site and the consequences of stray electrical currents.[4]

NEW BIPOLAR LIGATING-CUTTING DEVICES

The latest advances in bipolar electrosurgery arise from the evolution and development of instant feedback technology that delivers either pulsed or continuous electrical output with constant voltage by only moderating the output current. This new breed of electrosurgical generators is paired with a variety of novel ligating–cutting devices manufactured to provide continuous feedback about tissue impedance at the treatment site. By near instantaneous response to incremental changes in tissue resistance, total energy delivery using these newer devices is dramatically less than with conventional bipolar systems. Once tonal feedback from the generator signals complete desiccation of the tissue bundle, the pedicle is typically cut by advancing a centrally set mechanical blade. These devices should logically reduce tissue carbonization, sticking, plume, and lateral thermal damage. As a general rule, low-voltage bipolar desiccation of compressed vessels is more effective under reduced tissue tension. All are able to adequately seal blood vessels up to 7 mm in diameter.

To date, there are 3 innovative bipolar platforms that utilize low constant voltage and impedance feedback along with paired ligating–cutting devices. Having established that vessel wall fusion can be achieved using electrical energy to denature collagen and elastin in vessel walls to reform into a permanent seal, the LigaSure Vessel Sealing Device (Covidien, Boulder, CO, USA) applies a high coaptive pressure to the tissue bundle during the generation of tissue temperatures under 100°C; hydrogen cross-links are first ruptured and then renatured, resulting in a vascular seal that has high tensile strength. Similarly, the EnSeal Laparoscopic Vessel Fusion System (Ethicon Endo-Surgery, Inc, Cincinnati, OH, USA) desiccates by utilizing a set of thermoeleastic plastic jaws embedded with nanometer-sized spheres of carbon that conduct a locally regulated current and cuts by the advancing of a mechanical blade that squeezes the tissue bundle under very high pressure to create a coaptive seal and rapidly express tissue water. A third device, the Plasmakinetics Cutting Forceps (Gyrus ACMI, a division of Olympus Corporation, Southborough, MA, USA) delivers pulsed energy with continuous feedback control using conventional tissue grasping.

ELECTROSURGICAL TISSUE ENDPOINTS
Moderating Electrosurgical Tissue Effects: Current Density

The rate of heat production from the conduction of current in living tissue ultimately determines whether cutting or coagulation predominantly occurs. The rate of heat production is fundamentally linked to the concentration of current, known as current density. Practically speaking, manipulating electrode surface area (ie, the current density) ultimately determines whether coagulation or cutting predominates. Coagulation occurs whenever a larger electrode surface area is used in tissue contact, causing tissue dehydration, vessel wall shrinkage, and coagulation of blood constituents by slower tissue heating; on the other hand, a small electrode surface area in noncontact mode results in tissue cutting or vaporization by delivering a much higher density of current through sparking that rapidly superheats intracellular water (**Fig. 4**). In both instances, the type of current (ie, Cut vs Coag) or power setting (*W*) have little bearing on the net electrosurgical endpoint. In essence, the more concentrated the current, the more rapidly heat is produced. Consequently, higher current concentration is more effective and produces more heat per unit time. This explains why heat is concentrated at the active electrode and not at the substantially larger dispersive electrode during monopolar electrosurgery (**Fig. 5**).

The 3 fundamental types of electrosurgical phenomena—cutting, fulguration and coagulation —may be differentiated as being contact or noncontact in nature (**Fig. 6**).

Noncontact Phenomena: Cutting and Fulguration

Cutting/vaporization
The capacity to electrosurgically cut (vaporize) living tissue depends on the ability to deliver output current of sufficient current density. Electrosurgical sparking, the active ionization of the air gap between the active electrode and the target tissue, confines the current to a small strike zone and requires at least 200 volts of electromotive force. Because the cut, blend, and coag waveforms all satisfy this requirement, electrosurgical cutting can be accomplished using any of these output settings (**Fig. 7**).

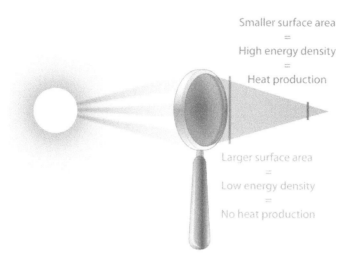

Fig. 4. Current density. During electrosurgery, the amount of current concentration, or current density, is determined by the size of the tissue area the current flows through (the surface area). (*From* Brill AI. Electrosurgery: principles and practices. APGO Educational Series on Women's Health Issues. Association of Professors of Gynecology and Obstetrics; with permission. Available at: http://www.apgo.org/electrosurgery/index.html.)

Using conventional electrosurgical generators, thermal damage at the margins of a cut is governed by the amount of voltage used. Decreases in current from progressive current interruption—cut to blend to coag—lead to greater output voltage ($V = I \times R$). With conventional electrosurgical generators, the higher voltages of blend and coag waveforms create progressively wider zones of thermal damage (**Fig. 8**) at the margins of the incision. These effects are amplified by using broad-surface electrodes and lower cutting velocity. Using blend or coag waveforms to cut to provide wider hemostasis can be helpful during myomectomy, for example, as well as when operating down the broad ligament and along the vaginal fornices during hysterectomy, or across vascular adhesions. Higher voltage outputs also facilitate incision of tissues with greater impedance, such as fatty or desiccated pedicles and adhesions. It is advisable to use the cut waveform via the edge of an electrode whenever lateral thermal spread may pose liability to adjacent tissues.[5]

Automatic feedback electrosurgical generators
Whereas the relative zone of lateral thermal necrosis of the cut margins is progressively greater when using the higher voltage outputs (ie, blend and coag) of conventional electrosurgical generators, newer units that employ impedance feedback provide more constant thermal margins regardless of the chosen waveform. Whereas the faster an electrode passes over or through tissue, the less thermal effects occur, newer automatic ESU technology that integrates feedback from the active electrode can deliver constant voltage to achieve the depth of coagulation, independent of the cutting rate. The active electrode can continuously monitor changes in the tissue impedance up to 4000 times per second and can adjust output voltage, current, and power every 300 microseconds. For instance, if 40-watt power output is selected, that output is delivered regardless of impedance change. This newer type of closed-loop controlled technology maintains the selected power setting

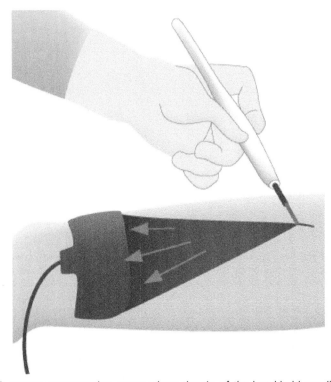

Fig. 5. High current concentration occurs where the tip of the hand-held pencil electrode is placed next to the skin. As the current travels through the body via the dispersive electrode, it is dispersed over a substantially larger surface area and is consequently less concentrated, precluding any clinical significant tissue effects. (*From* Brill Al. Electrosurgery: principles and practices. APGO Educational Series on Women's Health Issues. Association of Professors of Gynecology and Obstetrics; with permission. Available at: http://www.apgo.org/electrosurgery/index.html.)

despite variable tissue impedance by increasing the current output, not the voltage. This allows physicians to use lower power settings and to cause less thermal spread. Electrosurgical performance is markedly enhanced and the tissue product is more uniform and predictable.[5]

FULGURATION

Fulguration (superficial coagulation or spray coagulation) uses high-voltage sparking produced by the coag output to coagulate a broad surface with open vessels on end where coaption is not feasible or desirable. As opposed to the continuous arcing produced by the cut output, the highly interrupted coag output causes the arcs to strike the tissue surface in a widely dispersed and random fashion. With fulguration, sparks jump from 1 area to another randomly, "sprayed" rather than concentrated. High-voltage sparking results in high-temperature tissue changes, including carbonization; this technique leads to more rapid thermal change, creating a zone of superficial coagulation for fast control of bleeding across a wide area, such as oozing capillary beds or venous bleeding. Fulguration can be effective to control small bleeders up to 2 mm cut on end, such as along the

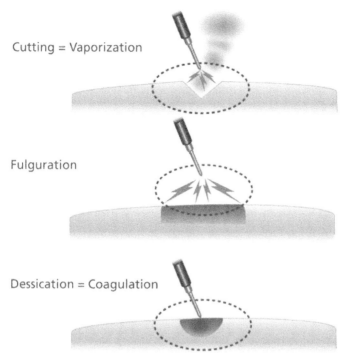

Fig. 6. Vaporization, fulguration, and coagulation are the primary triad of effects achieved via electrode manipulation. (*From* Brill AI. Electrosurgery: principles and practices. APGO Educational Series on Women's Health Issues. Association of Professors of Gynecology and Obstetrics; with permission. Available at: http://www.apgo.org/electrosurgery/index.html.)

undersurface of the ovarian cortex during cystectomy, and atop the myometrial bed during myomectomy.[5] Despite the high-voltage output involved, fulguration is ineffective in a wet, conductive surgical field owing to the widespread diffusion of current in blood.

ARGON-ENHANCED ELECTROSURGERY

Some electrosurgery generators use argon, an inert and noncombustible gas, as part of the current delivery system. At the active electrode, the emitted current is surrounded by argon gas. The current ionizes the gas; it becomes more conductive than air and provides an efficient pathway to the tissue. By definition, this technology is argon-enhanced fulguration. Because the beam concentrates the electrosurgical current, a smoother, more pliable eschar is produced. At the same time, the gas disperses the blood, ostensibly improving visualization. Because the heavier argon displaces some of the oxygen at the surgical site, less smoke is produced.[5]

CONTACT PHENOMENA: DESICCATION AND COAGULATION

Coagulation is a general term that includes both fulguration and desiccation (also called deep coagulation). Touching tissue with the surface of any active electrode, regardless of the selected waveform, obliterates any ionizable gap and leads to the diffusion of current with substantially lower current density. Consequently, the tissue

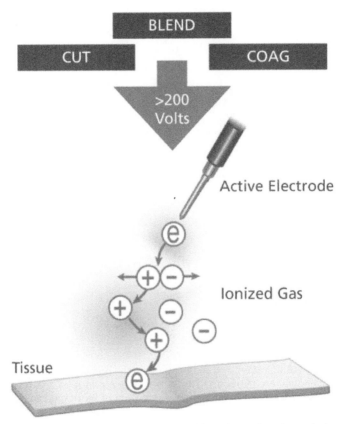

Fig. 7. Any waveform can be used for cutting. Holding the active electrode just above the tissue results in rapid expansion of intracellular fluid and cellular explosion, with resultant clean tissue division. (*From* Brill AI. Electrosurgery: principles and practices. APGO Educational Series on Women's Health Issues. Association of Professors of Gynecology and Obstetrics; with permission. Available at: http://www.apgo.org/electrosurgery/index.html.)

is heated more slowly, causing cellular dehydration by gradual percolation, rather than by the volumetric explosion by superheated steam that is produced with higher current densities (**Fig. 9**). Desiccation and coagulation can occur whenever an activated electrode comes into direct contact with tissue for a sufficient amount of time. Desiccation occurs as cells become dehydrated but still preserve their form. When intracellular temperature reaches 70°C to 80°C, protein denaturation occurs and a white coagulum forms. At 90°C, there is just enough heat to destroy tissue without carbonizing it, causing an effect between hyperemia and carbonization. Further heating leads to development of eschar—carbonized blood and tissue—that occurs when tissue is hyperheated. Because of its low conductivity, eschar buildup on an electrode induces higher resistance (impedance) levels. A higher voltage may then be needed to overcome the resistance to complete the circuit (recall, $W = I \times V$).[3] Correspondingly, clean electrodes require less power, are more efficient, and produce more predictable thermal tissue effects.

Compared with noncontact electrosurgical cutting and fulguration, which consume energy to ionize the air gap for sparking, contact desiccation heats tissue more

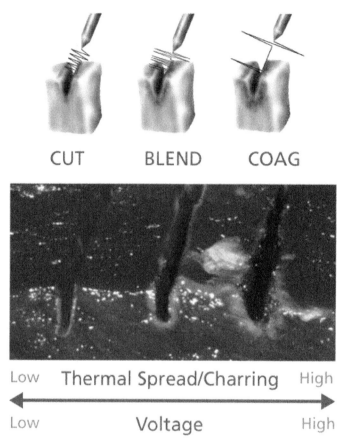

CUT   BLEND   COAG

Low   Thermal Spread/Charring   High

Low   Voltage   High

Fig. 8. Cutting can be accomplished using any of waveform, but the higher voltages of blend and coag create wider zones of thermal damage. Less coagulation effect occurs based on the shape and speed at which the electrode passes through tissue. (*From* Brill AI. Electrosurgery: principles and practices. APGO Educational Series on Women's Health Issues. Association of Professors of Gynecology and Obstetrics; with permission. Available at: http://www.apgo. org/electrosurgery/index.html.)

efficiently. Because there is more available energy to heat tissue, thermal damage is predictably deeper and more widespread during contact electrosurgical phenomena. When using the coag waveform, the peak voltage is very high, so contact coagulation using this waveform is generally limited to superficial layers. The high-voltage tissue strikes limit conduction in deeper layers by accelerating the buildup of tissue impedance from rapid desiccation and carbonization at the surface (see **Fig. 9**). Conversely, when using the lower voltage cut waveform, electrode contact heats tissue more gradually, leading to deeper and more effective penetration. Thus, both contact as well as coaptive coagulation using electrosurgery are predictably more effective using the cut waveform. For example, these precepts can help to determine the best waveform to electrosurgically ablate endometriosis. Because superficial-appearing implants may extend deeply into the retroperitoneal tissues, these types of lesions are best ablated using a broad-surface electrode in contact with the cut waveform. In contrast, superficial implants on the ovarian cortex may be more

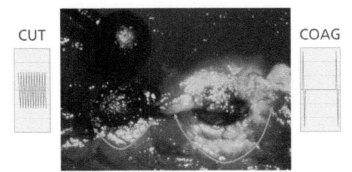

CUT   COAG

Fig. 9. Contact desiccation–coagulation. Varied tissue effects of different waveforms. (*From* Brill AI. Electrosurgery: principles and practices. APGO Educational Series on Women's Health Issues. Association of Professors of Gynecology and Obstetrics; with permission. Available at: http://www.apgo.org/electrosurgery/index.html.)

prudently treated using a smaller surface electrode in contact with the coag waveform to help minimize thermal injury to adjacent follicular tissue.

Coaptive vessel sealing with electrosurgery using any type of current may be ineffective if the blood flow remains uninterrupted. Unless a vessel is sufficiently squeezed before electricity is applied, the current density is significantly reduced by conduction in blood, and luminal temperatures undergo little change as any heat is dissipated by convection from the flow of blood. Directed by the appearance of a well-coagulated tissue pedicle, a fully pulsatile vascular core can be an unwelcome discovery at the time of surgical incision.

REDUCING RISK DURING CONVENTIONAL AND LAPAROSCOPIC ELECTROSURGERY
Electrosurgical Burns

A complicating factor in laparoscopic procedures is that most of the conductors, including part of the active electrode, are commonly out of the surgeon's field of view. Consequently, some injuries, such as burns to the bowel, may not be recognized immediately. Because it is possible to misdiagnose or be unaware of electrosurgical burns, the prevalence of complications resulting from laparoscopic monopolar electrosurgery specifically is likely underreported and underestimated. Prevention of these complications is of paramount importance, requiring the surgeon to remain vigilant when utilizing all electrosurgical instrumentation or techniques. Three types of stray current injuries are possible, especially during laparoscopic electrosurgery: Direct coupling, capacitive coupling, and insulation failure. All of these phenomena are more likely to occur with the use of high-voltage coag waveform. Using the lowest possible power settings (*W*) and the lower voltage cut waveform may help to reduce such risks.[6]

Direct Coupling

Direct coupling occurs when the user accidentally activates the generator (ESU) while the active electrode is near another metal instrument (**Fig. 10**). The secondary instrument becomes energized, and the energy seeks a pathway to complete the circuit to the dispersive electrode. Electrical sparks or arcing may be seen. If the pathway is via the viscera, and is of sufficient current density, unrecognized thermal injury may occur.[4]

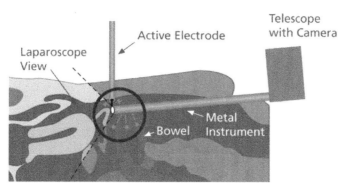

Fig. 10. Significant patient injury may occur if the generator is activated while the active electrode is located near another metal instrument. (*From* Brill AI. Electrosurgery: principles and practices. APGO Educational Series on Women's Health Issues. Association of Professors of Gynecology and Obstetrics; with permission. Available at: http://www.apgo.org/electrosurgery/index.html.)

Capacitance

Capacitance is the property of an electrical circuit to store energy. A capacitor exists whenever 2 conductors with different potentials are separated by an insulator. A difference of potential or voltage exists between 2 conductors that have differing numbers of free electrons (an overall negative charge on the conductor with excess, and a positive charge on the electron-deficient conductor). Although separation by an insulator prevents the flow of electrons between these conductors, the potential difference nevertheless creates an attraction or electrostatic force between them. This force results in an electric field and creates a reservoir of stored energy. When an AC flows through a circuit, the applied voltage and flow of current periodically changes direction. With each reversal of current flow, the energy of the stored electric field is discharged. Although no actual current flows through the capacitor, the charged current from capacitance completes the circuit and in essence conducts the AC. The amount of capacitance is directly proportional to the voltage (ie, lowest with the cut and highest with the coag waveforms).[4]

Capacitive Coupling

Capacitive coupling occurs when energy from an active electrode is transferred across the insulator surrounding it to another conductor,[3] such as to an outer trocar sheath of an electrosurgical instrument. Although there is an insulator between the electrode and the trocar sheath, an electrostatic field between the 2 bodies induces the current to flow through the insulation, momentarily moving current from the active electrode to the trocar sheath (**Fig. 11**). The localization of current during bipolar electrosurgery eliminates the risk of capacitive coupling during laparoscopic surgery and the propensity of current to seek alternate current pathways to ground.[4]

   If the trocar sheath is in direct contact with the abdominal wall, the induced charge is released by ready conduction to the dispersive electrode. However, if the sheath is isolated by a plastic collar or other insulated material, the charge remains isolated to the outer cannula as long as the electrosurgical generator (ESU) is on. If isolated, and if the current density is of sufficient magnitude, contact between the sheath and adjacent tissue such as the bowel can result in thermal injury—often outside of the surgeon's field of view.

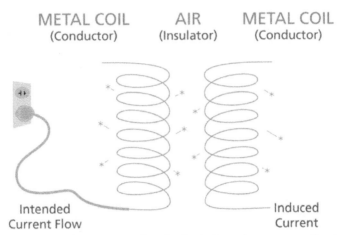

Fig. 11. An electrostatic field between the 2 bodies induces the current to flow through the insulation, momentarily moving current from the active electrode to the cannula. (*From* Brill AI. Electrosurgery: principles and practices. APGO Educational Series on Women's Health Issues. Association of Professors of Gynecology and Obstetrics; with permission. Available at: http://www.apgo.org/electrosurgery/index.html.)

Even if an all-plastic system is used, there is still a risk for capacitive coupling, because the patient's tissues can act as the second conductor. For example, if a patient's bowel is draped over a plastic trocar sheath, energy could travel by that pathway to body structures. The risk of capacitive coupling increases with longer instruments, thinner electrode insulation, narrow cannulas, and again, higher voltage waveforms.[4]

All surgeons have experienced an unexpected shock across his or her gloved fingers while stabilizing a clamp in contact with a monopolar electrode. Although many such burns occur from the direct conduction of concentrated current through the hydrated rubber or a hole in the surgeon's glove, these phenomena can also result from capacitive coupling. In the latter case, the electrified clamp and the surgeon's fingers are conductors with significantly different potentials. Activating the electrode, especially before contacting the clamp (generating higher voltage), induces a coupled current on the surgeon's fingers. If the area of contact between the fingers and the clamp is small, the current density will be high enough to generate a burn. Capacitance-induced burns across surgical gloves can be eliminated by avoiding open circuit (noncontact) activation and cradling the surgical clamp with a large surface area.

Insulation Failure

Insulation failure potentially produces an alternate current pathway (**Fig. 12**). The often-undetectable smaller insulation breaks are more dangerous than larger breaks, because of current concentration. Failure may occur as a result of normal wear and tear, microscopic imperfections, routine use of the higher voltage coag waveform, and repeated electrode insertion into a trocar. To reduce the risk of insulation failure, electrodes should undergo periodic assessment for excess wear and minimizing the use of high voltage levels associated with the coag and higher blend waveforms.

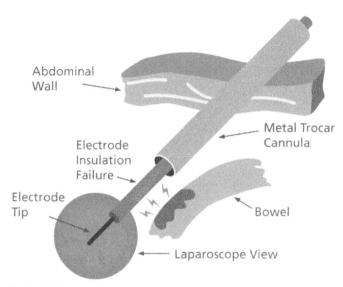

Fig. 12. Insulation failure can cause serious patient burns as well as staff injuries. (*From* Brill AI. Electrosurgery: principles and practices. APGO Educational Series on Women's Health Issues. Association of Professors of Gynecology and Obstetrics; with permission. Available at: http://www.apgo.org/electrosurgery/index.html.)

SUMMARY

Science becomes art and art becomes function when fundamental principles are utilized to dictate surgical practice. Most important, the risk for inadvertent thermal injury during electrosurgery can be minimized by a sound comprehension of the predictable behaviors of electricity in living tissue.

Guided by the Hippocratic charge of *primum non nocere*, the ultimate aim of energy-assisted surgery is the attainment of anatomic dissection and hemostasis with the least amount of collateral damage and subsequent scar tissue formation. Ideally, the surgeon's final view of the operative field should accurately approximate the topography discoverable after postoperative healing. Despite the continued innovation of products borne to reduce thermal damage and then marketed as being comparatively safer, it is the hands and mind of the surgeon that serve to preserve tissue integrity by reducing the burden of delayed thermal necrosis and taking steps to prevent excessive devitalization of tissue. Regardless of the chosen modality, the inseparable and exponentially linked elements of time and the quantity of delivered energy must be integrated while purposefully moderating to attain the desired tissue effect. Ultimately, the reduction of unwanted thermal injury is inherently linked to good surgical judgment and technique, a sound comprehension of the applied energy modality, and the surgeon's ability to recognize anatomic structures within the field of surgical dissection as well as those within the zone of significant thermal change. During the use of any energy-based device for hemostasis, out of sight must never mean out of mind. If the bowel, bladder, or ureter is in close proximity to a bleeder, they should be sufficiently mobilized before applying energy. Thermal energy should always be withheld until an orderly sequence of anatomic triage is carried out. Whenever a vital structure cannot be adequately mobilized, hemorrhage is preferentially controlled by using mechanical tamponade or suture ligature.

REFERENCES

1. Brill AI. Bipolar electrosurgery: convention and innovation. Clin Obstet Gynecol 2008; 51:153–8.
2. Harrell AG. Energy sources in laparoscopy. Semin Laparoscopic Surg 2004;11:201–9.
3. Wu MP, Ou CS, Chen SL, et al. Complications and recommended practices for electrosurgery in laparoscopy. Am J Surg 2000;179:67–73.
4. Brill AI, Feste JR, Hamilton TL, et al. Patient safety during laparoscopic monopolar electrosurgery-principles and guidelines. JSLS 1998;2:221–5.
5. Brill A. Energy-based techniques to ensure hemostasis and limit damage during laparoscopy. OBGMgmt 2003;15:5.
6. Brill AI. Energy systems in laparoscopy. In: A practical manual of laparoscopy & minimally invasive gynecology. London: Informa Healthcare/CRC Press; 2007. p. 86–9.

Uterine Leiomyomas, Current Concepts: Pathogenesis, Impact on Reproductive Health, and Medical, Procedural, and Surgical Management

Malcolm G. Munro, MD, FRCS(c)[a,b,]*

KEYWORDS

- Uterine leiomyoma • Uterine fibroids • Myomectomy
- Uterine artery embolization • Hysterectomy
- Abnormal uterine bleeding

Uterine leiomyomas are extremely common neoplasms that by the age of 50 are found in the uterus of almost 70% of white women and more than 80% of women of African ancestry.[1] Growth of leiomyomas is largely dependent on female gonadal steroids, especially estrogens and progesterone, and following menopause they spontaneously regress.

The majority of women who harbor leiomyomas do not experience symptoms such as infertility or abnormal uterine bleeding (AUB), leading to the conclusion that the vast majority of leiomyomas are asymptomatic. A corollary notion is that in the presence of symptoms such as AUB, infertility, pain, and pressure, identified leiomyomas may or may not contribute to the symptom complex. Therefore, faced with a patient with both symptoms and leiomyomas, it is incumbent upon the clinician to determine which if any of the leiomyomas contribute to the symptoms and which do not and are functioning as "innocent bystanders."

In the United States it is estimated that leiomyomas account for 30% to 40% of the approximately 600,000 hysterectomies performed annually, most of which are

Disclosures: Consultant for Aegea Inc, Bayer Healthcare, Boston Scientific, Ethicon Endosurgery, Ethicon Women's Health and Urology, Gynesonics Inc, Idoman Teoranta, Karl Storz Endoscopy Americas.

[a] Department of Obstetrics & Gynecology, David Geffen School of Medicine at University of California, Los Angeles, CA, USA
[b] Kaiser Permanente, Los Angeles Medical Center, Los Angeles, CA, USA
* Corresponding author. 4900 Sunset Boulevard, Station 3-B, Los Angeles, CA 90027, USA.
E-mail address: mmunro@ucla.edu

accomplished by laparotomy (66%),[2] an expensive and typically cosmetically impactful procedure that has substantial incumbent morbidity.[3,4] The last two decades have witnessed the development or increased use of procedures designed to reduce morbidity associated with leiomyoma-related therapy, ranging from hysterectomy without laparotomy (vaginal and laparoscopic hysterectomy) to less invasive and uterine-sparing interventions such as laparoscopic or hysteroscopic myomectomy, to image-guided techniques like uterine artery embolization and myoma ablation with cryotherapy, radiofrequency electricity, or focused ultrasound. Finally, whereas this article is included in a publication dedicated to less-invasive therapeutic procedures, it is important for the clinician to understand not only the known factors impacting growth and development of leiomyomas, but also the potential role of medical management of these highly prevalent lesions.

LEIOMYOMA GROWTH AND DEVELOPMENT

To understand medical therapy of leiomyomas requires some understanding of the myriad genetic factors and growth and steroid hormones that potentially influence leiomyoma development and growth. Unfortunately, estrogens have been perceived by many as the key, and even only stimulators of myoma growth, largely because the volume of a leiomyoma typically decreases following menopause. On the surface, this process seems to be simply related to hypoestrogenemia, even though the endocrinologic milieu of the postmenopausal woman is typified by other changes in the circulating levels of gonadal steroid hormones including the relative absence of progesterone. This relationship is particularly interesting in the context that progesterone receptor concentrations in leiomyomas are much higher than in normal myometrium. Progesterone has been demonstrated to upregulate factors associated with leiomyoma growth including Bcl-2 protein, proliferating cell nuclear antigen and epidermal growth factor.[5,6] There is evidence that progestins may result in growth of leiomyomata and that antiprogestational agents have the opposite effect.[7]

Other evidence exists for the role of progesterone in myoma growth. Gonadotropin-releasing hormone agonist (GnRH-a)–treated patients enter a temporary "medical" menopause, frequently requiring that estrogen and/or progestin add-back therapy be provided to treat vasomotor symptoms or vaginal atrophy and to protect against osteopenia. Women so treated have been subjected to randomized trials comparing progestin-only add-back to estrogen-progestin regimens. In most instances myoma growth or lack of volume reduction has been demonstrated only in association with progestin use and is not seen with estrogen-progestin therapy.[8] Another clue to the influence of progestins on myoma growth is that antiprogestational therapy has been demonstrated to reduce myoma volume in conjunction with reductions in progesterone receptor levels despite estradiol levels remaining normal.[7,9,10] All of these findings suggest that progestins play a significant if not dominant role in the growth of leiomyomas, and that estrogens are important, but in themselves, are unlikely to directly cause growth of leiomyomas.

Leiomyomas may be present in a number of locations in the uterus; features that have been incorporated into the design of the Federation International d'Obstetrique et Gynecologie (FIGO) classification system of causes of AUB in the reproductive years and called the PALM-COEIN system (**Fig. 1**).[11] The acronym is pronounced palm-coin, with each letter uniquely representing one of the classification categories. Generally, the PALM group represents entities that are currently clearly definable by gross and/or histopathologic evaluation. On the other hand, the COEIN group includes entities that are not definable structurally or histopathologically; they may occur in a structurally normal uterus. The one exception is the Not Classified (N)

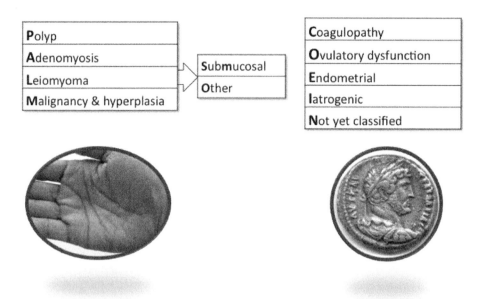

Polyp			Coagulopathy
Adenomyosis	Submucosal		Ovulatory dysfunction
Leiomyoma	Other		Endometrial
Malignancy & hyperplasia			Iatrogenic
			Not yet classified

Fig. 1. Basic FIGO classification system for causes of AUB in the reproductive years. The system includes four categories that are defined by visually objective structural criteria (PALM: polyp, adenomyosis, leiomyoma, malignancy or hyperplasia); four unrelated to structural anomalies (COEI; coagulopathy, ovulatory dysfunction, endometrial, iatrogenic); and one (N) that includes entities not yet classified. The leiomyoma category (L) is subdivided into those patients who have at least one submucous myoma (Lsm) and those with myomas that do not impact the endometrial cavity (Lo). When used in informatl notation, the letters AUB are followed by a hyphen in front of each identified entity - eg, AUB-P, -O denotes an individual with abnormal uterine bleeding in the presence of an endometrial polyp but that is also thought to occur in the context of an ovulatory disorder. (*Reproduced from* Munro MG, Critchley HO, Broder MS, et al. The FIGO classification system (PALM-COEIN) for causes of abnormal uterine bleeding in non-gravid women in the reproductive years, including guidelines for clinical investigation. Int J Gynaecol Obstet 2011;113:3–13; *with permission.*)

category that includes rare or ill-defined entities such as arteriovenous malformations and endometritis. The leiomyoma category is subdivided into SM or O, depending on the presence of at least one submucus leiomyoma when the subclassification of SM is applied, or O if all the myomas are either intramural or subserosal. A more detailed subclassification of leiomyomas is also included that builds on the already established system for describing submucous lesions originally published by Wamsteker[12] but adds categorization for the locations of leiomyomas that do not distort the endometrial cavity (**Fig. 2**). Use of this subclassification system should help better define research and discussion regarding both the role and treatment of leiomyomas in gynecologic disorders.

With regard to leiomyosarcoma, misperceptions of the risk of malignancy in leiomyomas may have a profound impact on the decision-making of women contemplating the spectrum of therapeutic approaches to their clinical problem. First, it is important for both clinicians and women to understand that leiomyosarcoma likely represents a de novo neoplasm and is not a result of malignant transformation of a benign tumor. Leiomyosarcoma is extremely rare, particularly in premenopausal

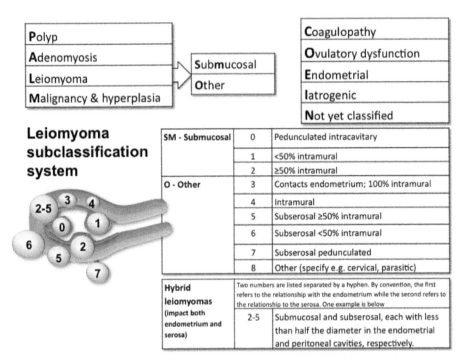

Polyp		Submucosal	
Adenomyosis		Other	
Leiomyoma			
Malignancy & hyperplasia			

Coagulopathy
Ovulatory dysfunction
Endometrial
Iatrogenic
Not yet classified

Leiomyoma subclassification system

SM - Submucosal	0	Pedunculated intracavitary
	1	<50% intramural
	2	≥50% intramural
O - Other	3	Contacts endometrium; 100% intramural
	4	Intramural
	5	Subserosal ≥50% intramural
	6	Subserosal <50% intramural
	7	Subserosal pedunculated
	8	Other (specify e.g. cervical, parasitic)
Hybrid leiomyomas (impact both endometrium and serosa)	Two numbers are listed separated by a hyphen. By convention, the first refers to the relationship with the endometrium while the second refers to the relationship to the serosa. One example is below	
	2-5	Submucosal and subserosal, each with less than half the diameter in the endometrial and peritoneal cavities, respectively.

Fig. 2. FIGO classification system including the leiomyoma subclassification. The classification of leiomyomas categorizes the submucous (sm) group according to the Wamsteker system[12] and adds categorizations for intramural, subserosal, and transmural lesions. Intracavitary lesions are attached to the endometrium by a narrow stalk and are classified as type 0, whereas types 1 and 2 require that a portion of the lesion is intramural with type 1 being 50% or less and type 2 more than 50%. Type 3 lesions are totally extracavitary but abut the endometrium. Type 4 lesions are intramural leiomyomas that are entirely within the myometrium with no extension to the endometrial surface or to the serosa. Subserosal (types 5–7) myomas include type 5, which are more than 50% intramural; type 6, which are 50% or less intramural, and type 7 being attached to the serosa by a stalk. Lesions that are transmural are categorized by their relationships to both the endometrial and serosal surfaces. The endometrial relationship is noted first whereas the serosal relationship is second (eg, type 2–5). An additional category, type 8, is reserved for myomas that do not relate to the myometrium at all and include cervical lesions, those that exist in the round or broad ligaments without direct attachment to the uterus, and other so-called parasitic lesions. (*Reproduced from* Munro MG, Critchley HO, Broder MS, et al. The FIGO classification system (PALM-COEIN) for causes of abnormal uterine bleeding in non-gravid women in the reproductive years, including guidelines for clinical investigation. Int J Gynaecol Obstet 2011;113:3–13; *with permission.*)

women, even in the context of rapid enlargement. It is more frequently encountered in the sixth or seventh decade of life in which it has been reported to occur in 1.4% to 1.7% of women undergoing hysterectomy.[13,14] For premenopausal women, understanding that a myoma is almost certainly benign should allow for the consideration of expectant medical approaches, minimally invasive procedures, or myomectomy, without undue concern for the presence of malignancy. However, for those women who are postmenopausal with a diagnosed enlarging myoma, malignancy is a distinct possibility, making medical or conservative surgical procedures inappropriate.

HOW DO LEIOMYOMAS CAUSE SYMPTOMS?
Abnormal Uterine Bleeding

The mechanisms involved in leiomyoma-associated AUB are only beginning to be understood. First, leiomyomas themselves are typically and strikingly solid and relatively avascular, so bleeding from the myoma itself is probably rare. On the other hand, the myoma may be surrounded by a relatively rich vasculature. When hysteroscopy demonstrates submucous leiomyomas (Lsm) in women with heavy menstrual bleeding (HMB), in most instances the tumors are covered by endometrium, whereas in others endometrium seems thin or even absent with a variable amount of perimyoma vasculature overlying the tumor.[15]

The search for biochemical mechanisms of leiomyoma-associated uterine bleeding has demonstrated a number of differences between myoma cells and normal myometrium. The smooth muscle cells that comprise leiomyomas release angiogenetic and growth factors such as vascular endothelial growth factor, basic fibroblast growth factor, and transforming growth factor (TGF-β) as well as plasminogen activators and inhibitors.[16] There is evidence from Yale University that TGF-β may have a direct impact on factors that impair local endometrial hemostasis.[17] It seems that when leiomyomas are adjacent to endometrium, elevated levels of TGF-β compete at the level of the endometrial stromal cell membrane for the receptor to a substance called bone morphogenetic protein-2 (BMP-2), which is normally responsible for the production in the nucleus of factors such as plasminogen activator inhibitor, antithrombin III, and thrombomodulin. The impact of reduced BMP-2 activity is a reduction in these substances and a corresponding impairment of local hemostatic processes in the endometrium.

Leiomyoma matrix metalloproteinase (MMP) 2 and 11 activity have been demonstrated to be increased, but MMP 1 and 3 remain unchanged. Unfortunately, the relationship of these findings to myoma-related AUB remains unclear.[18,19]

Still, the overwhelming clinical impression is that those myomas that cause bleeding are submucous in location and that the site of bleeding is usually the adjacent and/or overlying endometrium or, less commonly, the blood vessels that surround the tumor. This observation makes careful evaluation of the endometrial cavity important in determining the cause of AUB. Clinically obvious myomas, such as those detected by manual palpation, may have nothing to do with the bleeding, whereas submucous tumors not detectable on manual examination may be the responsible pathologic entity. Among the myriad questions facing investigators and clinicians is the role of FIGO type 3 lesions in the genesis of AUB.

Infertility and Recurrent Pregnancy Loss

Leiomyomas can be implicated in the genesis of infertility and early pregnancy loss, but not all myomas have this deleterious manifestation. A 2009 systematic review reported on the effects of leiomyomas on fertility and the performance of myomectomy on fertility and early pregnancy outcomes.[20] Of 347 studies initially evaluated, 23 were included in the data analysis but only four provided data that allowed evaluation of the impact of submucous fibroids (types 0–2) on fertility. The investigators concluded that women with submucous fibroids, compared with infertile women without such fibroids, demonstrated a significantly lower clinical pregnancy rate (four studies), implantation rate (two studies), and ongoing pregnancy/live birth rate (two studies).[20]

Further evidence regarding the impact of submucous myomas on fertility can be found in studies evaluating the fertility-related results of resectoscopic myomectomy.

It seems clear from high-quality trials that pregnancy rates are higher after myomectomy when compared with women undergoing no or placebo procedures.[20,21]

The mechanisms whereby submucous leiomyomas impact fertility are at the present time unclear. However, the Yale group has also produced high-quality evidence that such lesions may impart a global molecular impact that results in inhibition of the receptivity of the endometrium to implantation as determined by the presence of transcription factors such as HOXA-10 and -11. There seems to be a "field effect" that includes TGF-β–mediated reduction in the levels of endometrial HOXA-10 and -11 expression, both over the myoma, and remotely in the endometrium overlying apparently normal myometrium. Based on available evidence, this change is not seen in the endometrium of women with intramural or subserosal myomas.[17,22]

Whereas study of the impact of submucous leiomyomas on early pregnancy performance is difficult because of the multiplicity of factors potentially impacting early pregnancy loss, it seems likely that such lesions are associated with an increased risk of early pregnancy failure. In the metaanalysis of Pritts et al,[20] there were significantly higher spontaneous abortion rates in women with submucous leiomyomas (two studies, relative risk 1.68, 95% confidence interval 1.37–2.05, P = .022), a difference that seemed to be addressed by resectoscopic myomectomy.

The mechanisms by which submucous fibroids impair pregnancy outcomes remain unknown. Some investigators have reported that histologic examination of the endometrium overlying myomas[23,24] and opposite the fibroid[24] show glandular atrophy. Such a finding may be a histologically related manifestation of the biochemical impact of the submucous leiomyoma described by Rackow et al[22] reflecting a mechanism whereby implantation and nourishment of the developing embryo is impaired.

The Pritts et al[20] metaanalysis suggested that intramural myomas may have a role in the genesis of infertility or in in vitro fertilization success, but currently available evidence did not support the performance of myomectomy to improve fertility outcomes.[20] To date, studies have not been categorized by FIGO myoma type, leaving the possibility that there is a difference between outcomes and interventions associated with type 3 lesions and those that do not abut the endometrium (type 4 and greater).

Other Symptoms

If leiomyomas grow to the point of distorting surrounding structures they may cause a number of other symptoms that include pressure, urinary incontinence, and, less commonly, impact on bowel function.[25] Pain is another symptom frequently attributed to leiomyomas, and, for various reasons, sexual function may be adversely impacted. All of these symptoms can, and usually are caused by a plethora of other issues, a circumstance, given the prevalence of leiomyomas, that creates an opportunity for misdiagnosis of cause and effect. However, it is apparent that when leiomyomas achieve a threshold volume, bulk-related symptoms can substantially impact the quality of life for the woman. Unfortunately, there are few data evaluating the prevalence of these symptoms.

For years the author has told residents that when pain and leiomyomas coexist, pain is likely from another source, which some have called Munro's Rule. However, this rule was unencumbered by any evidence beyond the clinical experience of its author, and some studies seemed to suggest that leiomyomas and pain were related. However, such studies were hampered by an incomplete evaluation for other causes of pelvic pain, by evaluation based on ultrasound alone, and apparently not adequately considering other gynecologic and nongynecologic causes of pelvic pain.[26] Fortunately, attention is being paid in the literature to the putative relationship between leiomyomas and pain by analyzing for comorbid conditions. A retrospective case control study of women undergoing hysterectomy for leiomyomas demonstrated that those with concomitant adenomyosis were more than three times more likely to have pelvic pain including dysmenorrhea, dyspareunia, and noncyclic pain.[27] Another retrospective study demonstrated that of 131 patients who underwent laparoscopic myomectomy or hysterectomy, 113 had concomitant endometriosis, and those women who had both endometriosis and leiomyomas were more likely to have pain than those with leiomyomas alone.[28] These data suggest that Munro's Rule may have some legs and that when faced with a patient with leiomyomas and chronic pelvic pain, the clinician should be wary of ascribing the cause of the symptoms to the leiomyomas.

DIAGNOSING AND CHARACTERIZING LEIOMYOMAS

Because uterine leiomyomas are highly prevalent and frequently asymptomatic, it is important to both obtain a detailed and structured history and undertake a careful evaluation of the uterus before concluding that leiomyomas are contributing to the clinical problem. Just because there are symptoms and leiomyomas, the two are not necessarily related in a cause-effect fashion.

The diagnosis of leiomyomas is generally accomplished with one or a combination of hysteroscopy and radiologic techniques that may include transvaginal sonography (TVS), saline infusion sonography (SIS), and magnetic resonance imaging (MRI). The goal is to identify and characterize the lesions, distinguish leiomyomas from adeno-myomas, and identify those that are submucous in location. Lesions should be characterized as to the extent of myometrial penetration and the relationship to the uterine serosa because transcervical resection is not considered appropriate when the leiomyoma is close to or in contact with the serosal layer.

Leiomyomas Impacting the Endometrial Cavity

Given the notion that only submucous leiomyomas contribute to infertility, early pregnancy loss, and heavy uterine bleeding (AUB-Lsm), accurate determination of the relationship of myomas to the endometrial cavity is essential for patient counseling and treatment planning. Blind instrumentation has been demonstrated to be inade-quate for precise depiction of the structure of the endometrial cavity[29–31] when compared with any of a number of imaging techniques, including those that are ultrasound-based, and direct inspection with hysteroscopy.

There is a role for transvaginal ultrasound as a screening tool. In nonpregnant women with AUB, TVS showing an absence of myomas adjacent to or deflecting the endometrial echocomplex (EEC) is usually associated with a hysteroscopic examination negative for submucous leiomyomas. However, there is high-quality evidence from a Cochrane systematic review that demonstrates TVS to be still inferior to either SIS or hysteroscopy for the distinguishing intramural from submucous leiomyomas.[32] SIS is also known as sonohysterography or contrast sonography and is performed using vaginal ultrasound in conjunction with the transcervical instillation of a sonolucent substance such as saline, an approach that is comparable to hysteroscopy in its sensitivity for the diagnosis of intracav-itary polyps and submucous myomas.[33,34] Consequently, when ultrasound dem-onstrates myomas that exist suspiciously close to the EEC or when the EEC is deflected or difficult to evaluate, additional evaluation with saline infusion sonog-raphy or hysteroscopy should be considered.

Hysteroscopy is generally considered to be the gold standard of evaluation of the endometrial cavity for the presence of type 0 to 2 leiomyomas as well as other characteristics such as diameter and location (anterior, posterior, fundal, corneal, and so forth). Diagnostic hysteroscopy can usually be performed in an office environment, but unfortunately, at least in North America, relatively few clinicians seem comfortable with this approach, with most performing the procedure in a ambulatory surgery center or traditional operating room. A patient with a tortuous or stenotic cervix may be difficult to examine with office hysteroscopy, but most examinations can be performed successfully and comfortably with adequate and sufficient local anesthesia.[35]

MRI is another modality that has been shown to be accurate in the evaluation of the endometrial cavity in women with AUB. It is apparent that MRI is superior to either ultrasound or hysteroscopy at characterizing the relationship with the myometrium, including the serosa.[36] MRI has particular value in selected patients when neither SIS nor hysteroscopy are feasible because of virginal status or for women who have other issues with passing a device through the vagina.

Leiomyomas and the Myometrium

The myometrium is assessed to determine the extent of submucous myoma (type 0–2) involvement, to characterize types 3 to 6 leiomyomas, and to distinguish between leiomyomas and adenomyomas. Two-dimensional (2-D) TVS is generally useful for the evaluation of myomas in the myometrium, although variations in echogenicity can in some instances reduce the sensitivity of the examination. In addition, such 2-D imaging can be challenging when the mass comprising myoma and myometrium is large, because it is difficult to adequately image and track the various lesions identified. In such instances, three-dimensional (3-D) sonography may provide additional value.

Adenomyosis is a disorder characterized by endometrium or endometrial-like tissue within the myometrium. Although typically diffuse in nature, in some instances the disorder may be focal with lesions that have sonographic characteristics superficially similar to leiomyomas. In appropriately trained hands and with contemporary equipment, TVS is quite sensitive for the diagnosis of diffuse adenomyosis, and it approaches MRI in sensitivity.[37] However, there is less evidence evaluating the ability of TVS to distinguish focal adenomyosis (an adenomyoma) from leiomyomas, where MRI may be superior.[37] Color flow Doppler ultrasound helps to distinguish focal adenomyosis from leiomyomas because myometrial vessels course around the lesion, whereas in adenomyosis the vessels pass through the leasion retaining their vertical orientation to the endometrial cavity.[38]

MRI has been demonstrated sensitive in the evaluation of the myometrium for leiomyomas and is also effective at distinguishing them from adenomyomas.[39] MRI also seems superior to TVS, SIS, and hysteroscopy for measuring the myometrial extent of submucous leiomyomas.[36]

EXPECTANT MANAGEMENT OF LEIOMYOMAS

The process of watchful waiting is an option for most women with leiomyomas; however, counseling is difficult, in part because of variability in the natural course of any group or collection of tumors. The Fibroid Growth Study followed 262 leiomyomas in 72 women using sequential MRI scans over a period of 12 months. The median growth rate was 9%, but serially measured volume varied from an 89% reduction to a 138% increase.[40] Tumors in the same women grew at different rates, and whereas growth rates in black women and white women were similar under the age of 35, for women 35 and older the growth rate was much lower in white women. The growth rates for SM myomas were similar to those in other locations in the uterus.[41]

This information may be of value, for example, for the woman in the late reproductive years who has acceptable control of symptoms. She may choose to wait for menopause rather than undergo surgical therapy for her SM leiomyomas. Expectant management is more difficult for young women with, for example, intramural myomas (type 3 or 4), who are not currently in a position to try to conceive but who realize that their lesions may create symptoms and/or incrementally greater uterine damage with the passage of time.

MEDICAL MANAGEMENT OF LEIOMYOMAS

The use of medical therapy has expanded due to new information about the factors that affect myoma growth, the availability of new therapeutic agents, and a more reasoned understanding of the relationship of leiomyomas to symptoms. However, it is unlikely that these agents will have much of a role for women with infertility and AUB-Lsm because reduction (not elimination) of the structural distortion of the cavity is unlikely to result in improved fertility or pregnancy performance.

Gonadotropin-Releasing Hormone Agonists

The administration of gonadotropin-releasing hormone agonists (GnRH-a) results in amenorrhea secondary to the creation of a hypoestrogenic and hypoprogestogenic state. For women with leiomyoma-related symptoms, these agents may be used strategically in a number of ways that range from short-term courses in preparation for surgery to longer term use that may even preempt the need for operative intervention. GnRH-a administration results in a reduction of both leiomyoma and total uterine volume by a mean of about 50% by 12 weeks.[42] This outcome is temporary, however, because the volume of both the uterus and myoma return to baseline levels within a few months following the cessation of therapy. Although the use of GnRH-a is associated with the side effects of hypoestrogenemia, including vasomotor symptoms and vaginal atrophy, the only concerning adverse outcome is osteopenia if therapy is prolonged for more than 6 months.[43] This reduction in bone density can be mitigated with the use of so-called add-back therapy with an estrogen, selected types of progestins, or estrogen-progestin combination therapy.[44]

Short-term use (2–3 months) of GnRH-a, in conjunction with iron supplementation, provides an opportunity for the woman with AUB and associated anemia to reconstitute her circulating hemoglobin levels without resorting to either blood transfusion or emergency surgery.[45,46] By ameliorating fatigue, the woman has the opportunity to select long-term medical or surgical therapy in a less stressed environment. For women who have decided on an operative intervention, GnRH-a–induced amenorrhea is a way to defer surgery to a more convenient time.

There may be a lasting impact of GnRH-a therapy on women with AUB and leiomyomas. A study on women who had completed 6 months of GnRH-a, randomized to either placebo or medroxyprogesterone acetate, found that a majority (about 55%) of each group experienced an improvement in their bleeding for months following discontinuation of agonist.[47] This evidence suggests that GnRH-a may have prolonged therapeutic benefit in such women, making the use of intermittent courses a potential nonsurgical strategy for women in the late reproductive years. Unfortunately, the studies were not designed to truly determine the causes of the bleeding in that there was no attempt to identify the location of the leiomyomas. Consequently, many of these women without submucous lesions may have had, for example, AUB-O (ovulatory disorder) because it is suspected that type 3 to 8 lesions do not cause abnormal bleeding.

Using GnRH-a to reduce uterine volume may facilitate the performance of minimally invasive hysterectomy in selected patients. Stovall and colleagues[48] found that 80% of women scheduled for hysterectomy with uteri greater than 14 weeks in estimated volume at baseline were able to undergo vaginal hysterectomy if GnRH-a was administered for the 3 months immediately prior to surgery. Such an approach may also have merit in facilitating laparoscopic hysterectomy and even laparoscopic supracervical hysterectomy, the latter by reducing the time for laparoscopically-directed morcellation, although there have been no clinical trials evaluating this hypothesis. There also exist data that show reduced blood loss associated with abdominal myomectomy; however, the absence of a difference in the incidence of blood transfusions makes the use of GnRH-a in this setting of questionable value.[49]

The evidence is mixed evaluating the preoperative use of GnRH-a for reduction of the duration and risks of resectoscopic removal of submucous leiomyomas. Early studies suggested that systemic intravasation of the uterine distention media was less, surgical time was reduced, and the procedures were easier to perform.[50,51] However, in a nonrandomized but controlled trial comparing resectoscopic myomectomy with and without preoperative treatment for 2 months with GnRH-a, the operating time was significantly longer in the GnRH-a group: 57.6 min versus 40 minutes.[52] This outcome was suggested by the investigators to be secondary to GnRH-a–related contracted uterus and cervical stenosis. In two recently published RCTs, operating time was either unchanged[53] or significantly reduced[54] in the GnRH-a–treated population. Notably, systemic absorption of distention media was significantly reduced in the study that reported reduced operating times.[54] Review of these articles demonstrates that there were substantial differences in study design: one randomized women with type 1 and 2 myomas,[53] whereas the other excluded type 2 lesions, limiting the study population to patients with only types 0 and 1 leiomyomas.[54] Neither study showed a reduction in the incidence of incomplete excision or the need for further procedures, although one of the trials may have been inadequately powered to make such a conclusion.[53]

Surgery may be unsuitable for some women for a number of reasons such as existing comorbidity or because there have been multiple previous pelvic surgical procedures, which substantially elevate the risk of surgery. Some women may simply prefer medical therapy. In such instances, long-term GnRH-a may be attractive, particularly for those who are near the time of menopause. In such instances decisions should be made regarding the use of add-back therapy with estrogen or estrogen-progestin compounds.[44]

Progestins

There is no currently available evidence regarding the use of systemic progestins for women with AUB-Lo (AUB in the presence of leiomyomas that do not distort the endometrial cavity), but there is evidence that the levonorgestrel releasing intrauterine system LNG-IUS may be effective in selected patients. A prospective but nonrandomized clinical trial included women with AUB-Lo with a sonographically-determined uterine volume less than 380 mL but at least one type II submucous leiomyoma 5 cm or less and no type 0 or type 1 lesions greater than 3 cm.[55] The reduction in menstrual blood loss at 3, 6, and 12 months postinsertion reached 90%, comparable with that of a group of women treated in the same center using a thermal balloon, and expulsion rates were about 5%.

Another group evaluated the impact of the LNG-IUS on women with leiomyomas without determining the relationship of those myomas to the endometrial cavity. The study showed high efficacy but, given the absence of endometrial cavity evaluation, it is likely that the study included many with abnormal uterine bleeding secondary to endometrial causes.[56]

Further study is required, but it would seem that LNG-IUS is a reasonable option for women with modestly enlarged uteri and at least selected type 2 leiomyomas. However, for very enlarged cavities, the clinical impression remains that therapeutic efficacy is less and spontaneous expulsion more common.

Antiprogestins

The important if not critical role of progesterone in the growth and development of leiomyomas has been described in this article.[57–59] The selective progesterone receptor modulator (SPRM) mifepristone, 5 mg per day, has been shown to dramatically reduce or even eliminate the symptom of AUB while reducing the volume of leiomyomas by about 50%, with few side effects.[10,60,61] In earlier studies using higher doses of mifepristone, endometrial hyperplasia was occasionally seen, but this adverse outcome seems uncommon, if not rare, at the 5 mg dose. Larger scale clinical trials will be necessary to further elucidate the cost-effectiveness of this approach. It is anticipated that within the next few years there will be additional SPRMs that have similar impact on leiomyomas and bleeding symptoms.

Aromatase Inhibitors

Aromatase inhibitors inhibit the physiological conversion of androgens to estrogens in the ovary and in peripheral tissues and thereby have the potential to impact leiomyoma growth. Indeed, there exists high-quality evidence showing that aromatase inhibitors reduce myoma volume by a mean of about 50%.[62,63] A RCT from Iran showed that the aromatase inhibitor letrozole was superior to GnRH-a in reducing myoma volume without vasomotor symptoms.[64] That these agents have undergone large-scale long-term clinical trials as adjuvant therapy for women diagnosed with breast cancer makes them interesting options for selected patients. Larger scale trials of these agents and their utility in the treatment of abnormal uterine bleeding associated with leiomyomas (AUB-L) and bulk symptoms are anticipated.

PROCEDURAL AND SURGICAL INTERVENTIONS
Myomectomy

In 1845, Atlee[65] first reported removal of leiomyomas via laparotomy, traditionally called abdominal myomectomy. The principles of contemporary abdominal myomectomy were established by Bonney,[66] with his publication of 20 years of experience and amplified by his 1946 report of 806 cases. The low morbidity and mortality were remarkable, with only 2 deaths in the last 400 cases (overall mortality of 1.1%).

Like many surgical procedures that were introduced in the 19th and 20th centuries, abdominal myomectomy had not been subjected to rigorous clinical evaluation comparing it with expectant, medical, and other surgical approaches to the various manifestations of uterine leiomyomata. Fortunately there remains controversy regarding its value; there are gradually accumulating data regarding the utility of myomectomy, especially for the treatment of infertility.

In the latter part of the 20th century, the advent of operative endoscopy changed the spectrum of surgical options for the woman with symptomatic leiomyomas. The introduction of hysteroscopically-directed management of submucous myomas offered an option with dramatically reduced surgical morbidity.[67] Laparoscopic myomectomy also offered an approach with potentially lower surgical morbidity that the laparotomic approach.[68,69]

With the increased ability to perform myomectomy with minimally invasive approaches comes another question: When should myomectomy be offered or performed? Indications for myomectomy by any approach are currently being reevaluated as cost containment incentives, medical therapy, consumer pressure, and academic introspection combine to reinforce the long known fact that most myomas are asymptomatic and do not require treatment. Even in the face of symptoms, as previously discussed, it is prudent not to assume that patient complaints are caused by the myoma felt on examination or imaged on ultrasound.

Preoperative preparation and evaluation

Preparation for myomectomy is undertaken in view of the need of the patient to understand the procedure, considering the expectant, medical, and other surgical options. The patient should have a clear understanding of potential complications as well as the expected and possible degree of postoperative disability. The potential for unanticipated hysterectomy should be reviewed. All of this information should be documented in the clinical notes and the informed consent document.

Most would find it prudent to preoperatively confirm tubal patency (if the procedure is designed to preserve or improve fertility) and to obtain as much information as possible regarding the location and extent of the myomas using one or a combination of hysterosalpingogram, SIS, hysteroscopy, and MRI. Such information may help in the selection of incision sites and perhaps in determining the route of access. If there is clinical suspicion that the masses in the uterus represent adenomyosis, MRI imaging may be appropriate because in such instances, conservative surgery is unlikely to improve reproductive performance. Ancillary investigations should be performed as appropriate; however, a hemoglobin or hematocrit is essential. In addition, because of the potential for blood loss, the patient should be provided the opportunity for collection and storage of autologous blood, provided her hemoglobin levels and the time available before surgery permit.

The preoperative use of suppressive medical therapy with GnRH-a, as discussed previously, may be particularly important for those women who have AUB and associated anemia because creation of amenorrhea can be expected to facilitate the restoration of hemoglobin levels, provided sufficient amounts of iron are administered over an adequate amount of time.[45]

There is controversy regarding the impact of prelaparotomic myomectomy GnRH-a use on the ability of the surgeon to detect small myomas intraoperatively and on the subsequent risk of recurrence. One RCT suggested that surgeons were more likely to miss myomas when the patient was treated with GnRH-a, whereas another showed no such relationship.[70,71] A Cochrane systematic review of RCTs concluded that, in addition to improving both pre- and postoperative hemoglobin levels, preoperative GnRH-a also reduced both operating time and the rate of vertical skin incisions.[72]

Procedures

Resectoscopic (hysteroscopic) myomectomy. Resection and vaporization are resectoscopic techniques used to remove leiomyomata, with limitations related to the size, number, and location of the tumors, especially in the cornual region, and to the proportion of the tumor that is in the myometrium. In addition, the goals of the patient with respect to fertility are important, because optimal retention or enhancement of fertility may require complete excision of the myoma with maximum preservation of endometrial and myometrial integrity. Resectoscopic myomectomy is more likely to result in improved bleeding symptoms ($> 90\%$) than successful treatment of infertility (53%–70%).[73–75]

Preoperative imaging is important, not only to select appropriate patients for resectoscopic surgery, but also to plan the technical approach itself. Lesions that are totally within the endometrial cavity (type 0 and superficial type 1) and that are appropriately sized (generally ≤ 5 cm diameter) can generally be vaporized and/or excised with relative ease. However, for those lesions that penetrate into the myometrium to a substantial degree (deep type 1 and type 2 tumors), careful planning and substantial skill with the resectoscope are important requisites. The margin between the uterine serosa and the deepest extent of the myomas should be measured,[76] and if it is less than 5 to 8 mm, the author suggests that intraoperative ultrasound and/or laparoscopy may be necessary to prevent injury to extrauterine structures such as bowel.

In most instances resectoscopic myomectomy is performed in a standard operating room under appropriate anesthesia. The patient is positioned in the dorsal lithotomy position, the cervix dilated, and the resectoscope positioned with a suitable electrode and attached to an electrosurgical generator. The author typically uses a combination of dissection, vaporization, and removal of the residual leiomyoma with a Corson forceps. Resection of deep submucous myomas is more often associated with systemic absorption of substantial amounts of distending fluid, a feature that should be made clear to patients, because in such instances the procedure may have to be aborted and completed at a later time.[74,77]

Laparotomic myomectomy. Laparotomic myomectomy may be performed if there are many leiomyomas, if they are very large, or if they involve adjacent structures in a way not suitable for the safe conduct of laparoscopic technique. At laparotomy, there exist a number of approaches that may reduce blood loss, including preoperative GnRH-a, mechanical vascular tourniquets, myometrial injection of vasoactive substances, and careful dissection technique. Vascular tourniquets are applied after creating windows in the broad ligaments that allow straps (usually urethral catheters or Penrose drains) to be placed around the uterine isthmus, occluding the blood supply from the uterine arteries. The vessels in the infundibulopelvic ligaments can be occluded bilaterally with vascular clamps, thereby obstructing the blood supply from the ovarian arteries, but in practice the author rarely takes this step.[78,79] The vasoactive substance of choice is dilute vasopressin, 20 units in 60 to 100cc of normal saline, injected around the myomas, taking care to avoid intravascular infusion.[80]

Avoidance of posterior incisions may be important because they have been associated with a greater incidence of postoperative adhesions,[81] and it is prudent to apply microsurgical techniques including meticulous hemostasis, careful tissue handling, and the use of fine caliber suture on peritoneal surfaces. There is some information supporting the use of adhesion barriers over myomectomy incisions.[82,83] Unfortunately, no data exist evaluating the impact of adhesion barriers on fertility.

Morbidity at laparotomic myomectomy was recently reviewed in 128 patients operated on by 46 surgeons with varying amounts of training; a likely measure of procedure effectiveness, because it reports results from surgery performed by a spectrum of surgeons.[84] The average uterine size was consistent with 14 weeks gestation, and the average estimated blood loss was 342 cc. Five had blood loss in excess of 1 L, the transfusion rate was 20%, and 1 patient required intraoperative hysterectomy. Postoperative complications included wound infection (1), deep venous thrombosis (1), and postoperative fever.

Laparoscopic myomectomy. Laparoscopically-directed myomectomy is in some ways controversial, but it has been demonstrated to be effective in a number of observational studies,[85-89] and with selected patients and expert surgeons was associated with shorter hospitalization, faster recovery, fewer adhesions, and reduced blood loss.[90] However, the spectrum of myoma size and location, the difficulty with morcellation and removal, and the technical requirements for manipulation of needles and suture with which to close the uterine incisions make the procedure difficult to perform. Nevertheless, retrospective comparative studies[91] and available RCTs [92] suggest that in selected patients, fertility outcome is about 50% to 60% with both the laparoscopic and laparotomic approaches. Another outcome important to women undergoing myomectomy is pregnancy outcome. Currently available evidence suggests that patients selected for laparoscopic myomectomy and operated on by skilled surgeons will have similar pregnancy outcomes compared with those who have laparotomic myomectomy.[93]

A review of the advantages, limitations, and concerns regarding laparoscopic myomectomy may be useful. The principal potential advantage compared with the laparotomic approach is the reduction of both direct and indirect costs. The small abdominal incisions generally reduce the need for analgesia, allow nearly immediate mobilization and alimentation, and facilitate earlier hospital discharge, frequently on the same day of surgery.[94] In addition, the lack of a significant abdominal incision allows a faster return to economic productivity, thereby reducing the indirect cost of care.

Theoretically, the reduced need for packs and manual retraction would minimize tissue trauma and subsequent adhesions. On the other hand, multiple myomas cannot usually be removed through the same incision, and the surgeon loses the ability to palpate uterine tissue to detect smaller myomas. It is also more difficult to apply laparoscopic technique to myomas in problem areas such as those adjacent to the uterine arteries or the cornua, thereby preserving tubal patency. As is the case with any laparoscopic procedure, there are geometric limitations posed by the location of the instrument ports. In some instances it may be more difficult to reapproximate myometrial and serosal tissue, a feature that may enhance the development of adhesions and which may increase the risk of uterine rupture should pregnancy occur. Morcellation of the excised tumors is now facilitated by the development of efficient endomechanical morcellators.[95] All of these factors conspire to increase operating time, frequently offsetting the reduction in postoperative direct costs intrinsically associated with laparoscopic surgery.

Minilaparotomy (with or without laparoscopic assistance). Frequently, laparoscopically-directed technique is not feasible or appropriate for a component of the procedure such as dissection near the cornua.[96] In such instances, a relatively small suprapubic incision can be enlarged sufficiently to complete that portion of the dissection or other component of the procedure, often with externalization of the myoma and/or uterus. This approach can also be used primarily without laparoscopic assistance.

From a short-term perspective, myomectomy by minilaparotomy or laparoscopic myomectomy with minilaparotomy have similar short-term outcomes including time to discharge, postoperative pain, and return to normal activity, when each is compared with the standard laparotomic approach.[97] Consequently, for clinicians who are not experienced or skilled with laparoscopic myomectomy, minilaparotomy-based approaches may provide patients with many of the benefits of minimal access surgery.

Vaginal myomectomy. There are a number of instances in which removal of a leiomyoma can be performed vaginally. The most obvious situation is when a submucous myoma prolapses through the cervical canal so that it can be removed simply by transecting or avulsing the stalk. This removal is typically accomplished by grasping the myoma with a tenaculum or ring forceps and twisting it until the lesion becomes detached. Clinically significant bleeding rarely occurs. In many instances the procedure can be performed in the office or procedure room with no or local anesthesia or in some instances with systemically administered anxiolysis or anesthesia. There may be value to performing postprocedure transvaginal ultrasound or hysteroscopy to evaluate for the presence of additional lesions in the endometrial cavity.

For submucous leiomyomas that have not prolapsed through the cervical canal, vaginal myomectomy has also been described following dilation of the cervix with laminaria, which are natural (elm) or synthetic rods that osmotically absorb existing fluid and slowly dilate the canal.[98] Smaller myomas can be removed intact, whereas morcellation can be used to facilitate the removal of larger lesions.

Another approach is vaginal hysterotomy, a technique that the author uses, in which incisions are made in the cervix to facilitate removal, a procedure that is hidden in a report published by Goldrath[99] more than 20 years ago. This approach can be used for leiomyomas that are present in the lower uterine segment and extend to the cervical canal, a location that is extremely challenging to access resectoscopically. To facilitate the procedure, the urinary bladder is dissected from the cervix in a fashion similar to that used for vaginal hysterectomy. Then, anterior and/or posterior longitudinal incisions are made in the cervix and extended as high as necessary to allow access to the myoma and dissection from the uterus. The incisions are closed with full-thickness continuous delayed absorbable suture. The author usually performs a second-look hysteroscopic procedure 3 to 4 weeks later to dissect free adhesions that may occlude the canal. Although successful for bleeding, the impact of this approach on fertility has not been evaluated, so patients must be cautioned in this regard.

Uterine Artery Embolization or Occlusion

Uterine artery embolization (UAE) is the use of interventional radiographic technique to occlude both uterine arteries with polyvinyl alcohol microspheres positioned by a catheter passed through the right femoral artery.[100] The procedure is generally performed under conscious sedation over a time that typically ranges from 30 to 90 minutes. Immediate postprocedure pain is generally substantial, requiring institutional admission at least overnight, typically with a requirement for narcotic analgesia. In some instances this pain is experienced in conjunction with fever, nausea, and vomiting—a constellation of symptoms that has been termed *postembolization syndrome*. Complications are relatively infrequent but include, in addition to postembolization syndrome, misembolization of tissues that include the ovary, ureter, and other structures; infection that has been associated with severe sepsis; and, rarely, death. Randomized trials with short-term outcomes do demonstrate that UAE likely has lower morbidity than hysterectomy, but patients should expect the side effects mentioned earlier and a readmission rate of 5% to 10%.[101,102]

There is evidence that UAE is an effective long-term solution for most women who select it. In a relatively large study of 200 patients, HMB was substantially reduced in 87% of patients at 3 months and 90% at 12 months of follow-up.[103] In this same group of patients, the total uterine volume reduced by 27% and 38% at 3 and 12 months, respectively. By 5 years, 73% had continued symptom control with 13.7%

and 4.4% undergoing hysterectomy and myomectomy respectively.[104] Another US registry that includes more than 2100 women has reported high degrees of satisfaction with the procedure and 3-year postprocedure hysterectomy and myomectomy rates of 9.8% and 2.8%, respectively.[105] Perhaps the most extensive review of UAE has been published in 2004 by the Royal College of Obstetricians and Gynaecologists in the United Kingdom. In this analysis, 32 articles representing 25 series of cases reported mean uterine volume and dominant fibroid volume reduced 26% to 50% and 40% to 75%, respectively, at 6 months following the procedure and marked improvement in bleeding experienced by 60% to 90% of those treated.[106] Finally, the Cochrane review of the three RCTs concluded that UAE offers an option to hysterectomy and, in some instances, myomectomy; UAE is associated with reduced institutional stay and faster return to normal activities; and overall satisfaction was equal to that of hysterectomy. However, unscheduled visits related to pain, fever, and discharge were more common.[107]

The issue of fertility following UAE is still under investigation. It is clear that conception and successful term delivery can occur following UAE,[108–110] but what is not clear is the incidence of infertility and of myoma-related pregnancy complications. The literature is mixed regarding the impact of UAE on fertility and subsequent pregnancy; it is possible that the impact is minimal in this population that already has an increased incidence of infertility. However, there may be unknown or unexpected adverse events such as the excess of intraperitoneal adhesions associated with UAE, described in a case control study from McGill University.[111]

In summary, bilateral UAE seems to offer an option to women with AUB-L that may provide long-term resolution of symptoms without the need for traditional surgical interventions. The role of this procedure in women who wish to conceive is unclear and requires further study. Clearly, myomectomy is the more traditional approach and for those with intracavitary lesions is the most appropriate procedure especially for those with infertility or wish to preserve fertility.[112]

Localized uterine artery occlusion (UAO) using laparoscopically-directed techniques has also been described. The uterine vessels are occluded with electrodesiccation or clips without the need for embolization. A number of series have been published with results similar to those available for UAE.[112,113] Two prospective comparative trials have demonstrated that clinical results may be similar and that patients undergoing UAO seem to experience much less pain than patients who are treated with embolization.[114,115] In a double-blind RCT from the author's institution, procedure-related outcomes of localized UAO using coils deposited in the uterine arteries by a fluoroscopically-guided catheter were superior to traditional UAE with microspheres.[116] The UAO patients had little procedure-related pain and could be discharged home the same day. Longer term studies are needed, however, to evaluate the comparative clinical outcomes of the two techniques.

Hysterectomy

As noted in the introduction, of the approximately 600,000 hysterectomies performed each year in the United States, a large proportion are performed for leiomyomas of the uterus.[2,117] The technical aspects of hysterectomy are discussed elsewhere in this issue.

It is clear that if total hysterectomy is to be performed and if it can be accomplished vaginally, vaginal hysterectomy is the preferred route from the perspective of cost, morbidity, and cosmetic result. The problem arises when vaginal hysterectomy is not feasible or is beyond the skill set of the operating surgeon. In such circumstances and with the advent of electromechanical laparoscopic morcellators and vaginal morcellating techniques, laparoscopic total and supracervical hysterectomy may be the only practical alternative to total abdominal hysterectomy for management of uteri with very large leiomyoma volume. Appropriate selection of patients excludes those without known or suspected preinvasive or invasive cervical and endometrial neoplasia.

Investigative Surgical Approaches

Leiomyoma ablation or myolysis

Techniques designed to destroy rather than remove leiomyomas have been termed *myolysis* or *myoma ablation*. Several such techniques are under development using liquid nitrogen for hypothermic ablation, laser or radiofrequency electricity, and, more recently, focused ultrasound energy, directed and monitored by ultrasound or MRI for hyperthermic ablation. These approaches have shown some promise, but well-designed clinical trials are necessary not only to determine their efficacy but, even if efficacious, to compare them with other techniques for clinically relevant outcomes.

Hypothermic leiomyoma ablation. The first publication of hypothermic treatment of leiomyomas was from the Yale group in New Haven, Connecticut, in 1996.[118] The technique, sometimes called cryomyolysis, uses probes cooled either by liquid nitrogen or by differential gas exchange, as described by Joule-Thompson. The probe is passed into a leiomyoma and then activated, resulting in a reduction of local temperature to less than $-90°$ C, creating an ice ball, the size and shape reflecting features of the probe and the duration of application. Lethal tissue damage occurs at $-20°$ C, but at the edge of the ice ball the tissue temperature is approximately $0°$ C and consequently is not destructive to the tissue.[119] A potential advantage of this technique over hyperthermic approaches is the ability to predict the limits of treated tissue by simultaneously imaging the ice ball with ultrasound.

The extent of tissue necrosis may be secondary to the degree of vascular damage. When tissue cools, the damaged vascular endothelium detaches from the internal surface of the vessel, a process that contributes to the development of edema and local activation of platelets. The resulting thrombosis then occludes the local circulation, thereby enhancing both local ischemia and tissue necrosis. The result is a graded response as histopathologic examination shows complete necrosis in the central aspects of the target area and tissue sparing in the periphery of the previously frozen tissue. The relative uniformity of cell death in the zones that reach $-20°$ C or lower suggests that the principal clinical impact of cryomyolysis is one that is secondary to the vascular impact on tissue.[119] There is also evidence that leiomyomata may be more sensitive to freezing than normal myometrial tissue, whereas the effects of laser or radiofrequency electrical energy are similar in myoma and adjacent healthy myometrium.[120] If this evidence is accurate, hypothermic ablation techniques may have a degree of tissue specificity and could aid the clinician in preserving neighboring myometrium.

In its present but experimental form, the technique is performed laparoscopically, usually under general anesthesia, with the telescope inserted through the umbilicus, or higher in the event of a large uterus. After exposure of the cervix with a speculum or retractors, a uterine manipulator is positioned and used to stabilize and manipulate the uterus, thereby optimally positioning the myomas for insertion of the probe (cryoprobe). The surgeon also positions additional ports, as required, for the instrument access necessary to perform the procedure. The location and number are determined at the time of the procedure based on the size and location of the myomas to be treated. An incision in the uterus, over the leiomyoma, is made with a monopolar electrosurgical hook or blade to create a passageway that is 4 to 5 mm wide and about 1 cm deep or less from the estimated inferior surface of the myoma. For myomas 4 cm or less in diameter a single central incision is adequate, whereas for larger diameter lesions multiple incisions will be required. The cryoprobe is then passed through the appropriate ancillary port and inserted into the myoma via the previously created tunnel. For larger myomas it is thought useful to reduce the blood supply from both the serosa and the endometrial vessels. Consequently, there exists a strategy of freezing the myoma superficially and then deeply using additional incisions, the number determined by the myoma volume.[121–124]

There are a number of studies evaluating this technique. In most instances both myoma volume and related symptoms, including HMB, are reduced by approximately 50% at 6 months and even more at 12 months following therapy.[121,123–125] These data are encouraging in that they suggest that hypothermic ablation is potentially a minimally invasive, safe, and feasible procedure in selected patients, There remain a number of questions including the effect of hypothermic ablation on fertility and future pregnancy, although a recent small series of 9 patients demonstrated that such patients may remain fertile and have essentially normal pregnancy outcomes.[126]

It is clear that these studies are insufficient to demonstrate long-term outcomes and that further studies with larger sample size and longer follow-up are needed to confirm the preliminary data. As a result, hypothermic ablation or cryomyolysis should still be considered an experimental procedure.

Hyperthermic leiomyoma ablation by laser and radiofrequency electrical energy. In the early 1990s coagulation of leiomyomas was reported under laparoscopic guidance using either laser (neodymium-doped yttrium aluminium garnet [Nd:YAG] or infrared) energy[127–129] or a bipolar radiofrequency (RF) electrical probe.[130,131] The energy from these different kinds of electromagnetic waveforms is converted first to mechanical energy, oscillating intracellular protein, then to the elevation of intracellular temperature that causes coagulative necrosis and resulting devascularization within the treated tissue. The volume of necrosis created is dependent on the amount of electromagnetic energy delivered to the tissue. There remain challenges related to predicting or monitoring the local distribution of this energy in tissue, although probes/electrodes with thermal couples that measure local temperature have some promise.

Hyperthermic myoma ablation is an investigational procedure that has been described via laparoscopy, hysteroscopy, and under ultrasound direction. When the procedure is performed laparoscopically, the laser fiber, monopolar or bipolar electrode is passed through the instrument channel of an operating laparoscope or ancillary cannulas and used to pierce the myoma and advance into its core. An attempt is made to coagulate the entire myoma by repeated insertions at multiple concentric sites. A few investigators have described the use of hysteroscopically-directed application of laser energy to ablate myomas or the portions of type 1 or 2 myomas that remain in the myometrium. The Nd:YAG fiber is guided through the instrument channel of an operating hysteroscope and positioned in the intramural myoma.[129] Unfortunately, positioning such a fiber without being able to view the uterine serosal surface is a concern. As a result, there is also some work under way evaluating the potential role of ultrasound-directed positioning of RF electrodes for the purpose of electrosurgical leiomyoma ablation, but no data are yet available.[132]

There are some outcome data available for laparoscopic hyperthermic myoma ablation. Typically there is a decrease in myoma volume within 6 months of up to 50% of the original size.[128–131] There is also evidence of reduction in the volume of HMB, but in the study with the largest sample size, it is unclear how much of this reduction is related to concomitant hysteroscopically-directed treatment.[131] Postablation pregnancy is a lingering concern because a number of investigators have reported adverse outcomes such as rupture of the uterus.[133,134]

Hyperthermic leiomyoma ablation by focused ultrasound energy. The potential for treatment of uterine leiomyomas using high-intensity focused ultrasound (HIFU) was first described in a multicenter feasibility study in 2003.[135] Focusing ultrasound energy essentially with a parabolic mirror for the ablation of tissue is a noninvasive technique first described in 1927 and then again in 1942.[136] The technique was slow to develop because of limitations in the control of the process of coagulative necrosis. With improvements in real-time imaging including ultrasound and MRI have come the potential for use of HIFU as a viable therapeutic instrument. Magnetic resonance-guided focused ultrasound surgery (MRgFUS) has now been evaluated in a number of tissues including breast,[137] brain,[138] and prostate gland.[139] Under development is the use of ultrasound for the direction of focused ultrasound energy.[132,140]

The treatment of uterine leiomyomas is performed in a specially designed suite with the patient positioned on a procedure table overlying the ultrasound generator. This system functions to create an array of pulsed high-intensity ultrasound beams that are focused on the target tissue, directed by MRI or possibly ultrasound imaging. One such array generates a volume of tissue ablation in the range of 6 mm by 25 mm using 2-D measurements. The device is then refocused to an adjacent target and the process repeated until the desired volume of tissue ablation is reached. Tumor necrosis is also dependent on the time of exposure. With MRI, the degree of tumor necrosis can to a degree be estimated, allowing the ability to thermally map the region of the target tissue to a prespecified temperature as measured by the proton resonance frequency shift.[141,142] However, preliminary studies comparing MRI-based treatment volume with the volume of nonperfused or necrotic tissue based on postprocedure hysterectomy and histologic examination reveal that the volume of myoma or myometrial necrosis is three-fold higher than that predicted by MRI.[143]

For uterine leiomyomas, the currently available data are almost totally derived from MRgFUS techniques. The patient is treated in an MRI suite where she is placed in the prone position with the abdomen resting over the treatment device. Conscious sedation is generally administered with a variable combination of narcotics and anxiolytics. The focused ultrasound unit is a spherically curved radiator contained within a sealed water bath. MRI is performed to ensure that bladder and bowel are not in the path of the ultrasound beams, and if so, manipulation or repositioning of the patient is done in an attempt to remedy the situation. Treatment, called *sonication*, is performed in a systematic fashion with typical treatment times to date being about 2 hours and time in the suite about 3 hours. Patients are discharged home about 1 hour following the end of the procedure.

The first published clinical study was a seven-center multinational multiinstitutional trial that described a series of 109 patients treated with the ExAblate 2000 system (InSightec, Haifa, Israel).[144] The mean fibroid volume of these patients, depending on the number of myomas, was 294 to 346 cm^3, whereas the mean treatment volume was only 32 to 36 cm^3, or about 10% to 11% of the total. There were relatively few treatment-related serious outcomes, but only 79.3% of the patients were available for follow-up at 6 months. The mean fibroid volume reduction was 13.5% $\pm$ 32 and, using the multidimensional Uterine Fibroid Symptoms and Quality of Life Questionnaire (UFS-QOL), there was a mean 27.3-point reduction in the score compared with baseline.

In a subsequent study and one that resulted in US Food and Drug Administration approval of a the ExAblate 2000 device for use in the United States, 109 of 176 women enrolled were treated in seven sites in the United States, Europe, and Israel.[145] In this trial the mean uterine volume was 595.0 $\pm$ 362.5 cm^3, the mean myoma volume was 284.7 $\pm$ 225.4 cm^3, and the mean treated myoma volume as estimated by MRI was 25.6 $\pm$ 18.4 cm^3. Several mild skin burns resulted, and 1 patient had a sciatic nerve injury that had resolved by the 12-month evaluation. The mean reduction in UFS-QOL was 23.8, and at 12 months with only 82 of the original cohort available for evaluation, 51.2% of the women reached the targeted reduction of at least 10 points.

More recently and in a well-designed comparative trial, the preprocedural use of GnRH-a has been shown to potentiate the effect of focused ultrasound energy as measured by intraprocedural MRI.[146] In a subsequent reported clinical series evaluating 49 women and followed for 12 months, UFS-QOL reductions of 45% were seen at 12 months, and 83% achieved at least a 10-point reduction in the scale.[147] The reduction in targeted myoma volume was 37% at 12 months in the patients available for evaluation.

The clinical results associated with MRgFUS are promising, but both myoma reduction and the measured relief of symptoms seem disproportionate to the amount of myoma treated. The feasibility study previously discussed demonstrated that the volume of tumor necrosis exceeded the treated volume by a factor of three. More recently a retrospective comparison was published comparing predicted volume of treated tissue, treatment volume based on MRI-determined temperature elevation, and MRI-determined volume of post treatment nonperfused tissue.[148] In this comparison, and only in larger areas of sonication, the volume of nonperfused tissue was double that of the treated volume based on MRI-measured tissue temperature. The investigators suggest that this larger area of necrotic tissue was caused by vascular occlusion and "downstream" ischemia, but the possibility exists that MRI is not as accurate as thought for the determination of treated tissue in these lesions.

Despite the apparent promise of leiomyoma ablation, there are still no published trials comparing any of the three procedures with experimental or established approaches such as UAE or occlusion, medical therapy, myomectomy, or hysterectomy. Indeed, some patients who have symptoms related to type 2 myomas may be candidates for endometrial ablation by any of a number of techniques. Furthermore, although the impact of myoma ablation on fertility and pregnancy is unknown, the few adverse outcomes reported following hyperthermic ablation with MRgFUS must be reason for concern. It is also clear that a number of patient characteristics including myoma size, location, and the presence of adhesions or abdominal scarring may to a greater or lesser extent impact or even preclude some patients from undergoing myoma ablation.

MRI- or ultrasound-guided FUS are the only techniques that have to date delivered energy to tissue without direct contact by the energy source with the treated tissue. Consequently, this approach offers the potential for incisionless surgery, at least for the selected patients who would qualify for therapy. However, the issue of prediction of the treatment volume must remain an area for concern given the structures that surround the uterus and the possibility for injury.

Despite all of the aforementioned reservations, these seem to be promising techniques to reduce the invasiveness of traditional surgery. The procedures should be subjected to appropriately designed clinical trials that can better define their role in the management of the myriad clinical circumstances associated with uterine leiomyomas.

For the present, the techniques must still be considered experimental and should be performed in a structured environment by well-experienced groups with patients carefully selected and counseled considering all available options. Careful observation and reporting of all results, both positive and negative, will help to define the role that myoma ablation has in the management of symptoms, including AUB, related to uterine leiomyomas.

SUMMARY

Leiomyomas are such common tumors of the uterus that at least two-thirds of women will have at least one by the age of 50. Despite this high incidence, we know relatively little about their cause, growth and development, and contribution to the genesis of reproductive disorders. The prevalence of lesions puts women with associated but unrelated symptoms at risk for unnecessary and/or unsuccessful interventions, especially if they have not been carefully evaluated and counseled. Indeed, because the majority of leiomyomas do not cause symptoms, when a woman presents with AUB, infertility, pelvic pain, or vague abdominal complaints, it is possible if not likely that the cause of the problem exists elsewhere. The other overwhelming impression that can be gleaned is this: when leiomyomas are the cause of the symptoms, particularly in women desiring to preserve fertility, the tumors have already and frequently induced irreparable harm, a circumstance that cries out for a strategy of early detection and interventions designed to minimize morbidity.

Fortunately, because of the efforts of a few, we are just beginning to understand the potential molecular mechanisms by which leiomyomas may contribute to reproductive tract symptoms such as AUB, infertility, and pregnancy loss, work that may contribute to the development of more specific medical therapeutic techniques and strategies. The use of increasingly precise and accessible imaging for diagnosis, combined with the application of customized intrauterine drug-releasing systems or minimally invasive and highly accurate targeted ablative technologies that minimize collateral damage, may provide women the opportunity to avoid the mutilating, painful, expensive, and frequently unsuccessful surgical interventions of today that are applied to end-stage disease.

For the present, clinicians should evaluate any woman with reproductive tract symptoms and leiomyomas carefully and with skepticism, ensuring that they have done all that is necessary to determine if the lesion or lesions are related to the problem. If leiomyomas are the suspected or known cause, clinicians must also be prepared to offer or otherwise provide access to the complete spectrum of care that the patient deserves, regardless of the limitations of the clinician's training, experience, or institutional environment. Such an approach will limit the number of unnecessary and ineffective interventions and, it is hoped, minimize morbidity while optimizing quality of life for affected women.

REFERENCES

1. Day Baird D, Dunson DB, Hill MC, et al. High cumulative incidence of uterine leiomyoma in black and white women: ultrasound evidence. Am J Obstet Gynecol 2003;188:100–7.
2. Wu JM, Wechter ME, Geller EJ, et al. Hysterectomy rates in the United States, 2003. Obstet Gnecol 2007;110:1091–5.
3. Carlson KJ, Miller BA, Fowler FJ Jr. The Maine Women's Health Study: I. Outcomes of hysterectomy. Obstet Gynecol 1994;83:556–65.

4. Garry R, Fountain J, Mason S, et al. The eVALuate study: two parallel randomised trials, one comparing laparoscopic with abdominal hysterectomy, the other comparing laparoscopic with vaginal hysterectomy. BMJ 2004;328:129.

5. Shimomura Y, Matsuo H, Samoto T, et al. Up-regulation by progesterone of proliferating cell nuclear antigen and epidermal growth factor expression in human uterine leiomyoma. J Clin Endocrinol Metab 1998;83:2192–8.

6. Yin P, Lin Z, Cheng YH, et al. Progesterone receptor regulates Bcl-2 gene expression through direct binding to its promoter region in uterine leiomyoma cells. J Clin Endocrinol Metab 2007;92:4459–66.

7. Murphy AA, Kettel LM, Morales AJ, et al. Regression of uterine leiomyomata in response to the antiprogesterone RU 486. J Clin Endocrinol Metab 1993;76:513–7.

8. Friedman AJ, Daly M, Juneau-Norcross M, et al. Long-term medical therapy for leiomyomata uteri: a prospective, randomized study of leuprolide acetate depot plus either oestrogen-progestin or progestin 'add-back' for 2 years. Hum Reprod 1994; 9:1618–25.

9. Steinauer J, Pritts EA, Jackson R, et al. Systematic review of mifepristone for the treatment of uterine leiomyomata. Obstet Gynecol 2004;103:1331–6.

10. Fiscella K, Eisinger SH, Meldrum S, et al. Effect of mifepristone for symptomatic leiomyomata on quality of life and uterine size: a randomized controlled trial. Obstet Gynecol 2006;108:1381–7.

11. Munro MG, Critchley HO, Broder MS, et al. The FIGO classification system (PALM-COEIN) for causes of abnormal uterine bleeding in non-gravid women in the reproductive years, including guidelines for clinical investigation. Int J Gynaecol Obstet 2011;113:3–13.

12. Wamsteker K, Emanuel MH, de Kruif JH. Transcervical hysteroscopic resection of submucous fibroids for abnormal uterine bleeding: results regarding the degree of intramural extension. Obstet Gynecol 1993;82:736–40.

13. Leibsohn S, d'Ablaing G, Mishell DR Jr, et al. Leiomyosarcoma in a series of hysterectomies performed for presumed uterine leiomyomas. Am J Obstet Gynecol 1990;162:968–74 [discussion: 74–6].

14. Parker WH, Fu YS, Berek JS. Uterine sarcoma in patients operated on for presumed leiomyoma and rapidly growing leiomyoma. Obstet Gynecol 1994;83:414–8.

15. Patterson-Keels LM, Selvaggi SM, Haefner HK, et al. Morphologic assessment of endometrium overlying submucosal leiomyomas. J Reprod Med 1994;39:579–84.

16. Stewart EA, Nowak RA. Leiomyoma-related bleeding: a classic hypothesis updated for the molecular era. Hum Reprod Update 1996;2:295–306.

17. Sinclair DC, Mastroyannis A, Taylor HS. Leiomyoma simultaneously impair endometrial BMP-2-mediated decidualization and anticoagulant expression through secretion of TGF-beta3. Journal Clin Endocrinol Metab 2011;96:412–21.

18. Palmer SS, Haynes-Johnson D, Diehl T, et al. Increased expression of stromelysin 3 mRNA in leiomyomas (uterine fibroids) compared with myometrium. J Soc Gynecol Investig 1998;5:203–9.

19. Bogusiewicz M, Stryjecka-Zimmer M, Postawski K, et al. Activity of matrix metalloproteinase-2 and -9 and contents of their tissue inhibitors in uterine leiomyoma and corresponding myometrium. Gynecol Endocrinol 2007;23:541–6.

20. Pritts EA, Parker WH, Olive DL. Fibroids and infertility: an updated systematic review of the evidence. Fertil Steril 2009;91:1215–23.

21. Shokeir T, El-Shafei M, Yousef H, et al. Submucous myomas and their implications in the pregnancy rates of patients with otherwise unexplained primary infertility undergoing hysteroscopic myomectomy: a randomized matched control study. Fertil Steril 2010;94:724–9.

22. Rackow BW, Taylor HS. Submucosal uterine leiomyomas have a global effect on molecular determinants of endometrial receptivity. Fertil Steril 2010;93:2027–34.
23. Deligdish L, Loewenthal M. Endometrial changes associated with myomata of the uterus. J Clin Pathol 1970;23:676–80.
24. Maguire M, Segars JH. Benign uterine disease: leiomyomata and benign polyps. In: Aplin JD, editor. The endometrium: Molecular, cellular and clinical perspectices. 2nd edition. London: Informa Health Care; 2008.
25. Stewart EA. Uterine fibroids. Lancet 2001;357:293–8.
26. Lippman SA, Warner M, Samuels S, et al. Uterine fibroids and gynecologic pain symptoms in a population-based study. Fertil Storil 2003;80:1488 94.
27. Taran FA, Weaver AL, Coddington CC, et al. Characteristics indicating adenomyosis coexisting with leiomyomas: a case-control study. Human Reprod 2010; 25:1177–82.
28. Huang JQ, Lathi RB, Lemyre M, et al. Coexistence of endometriosis in women with symptomatic leiomyomas. Fertil Steril 2010;94:720–3.
29. Valle RF. Hysteroscopic evaluation of patients with abnormal uterine bleeding. Surg Gynecol Obstet 1981;153:521–6.
30. Gimpelson RJ, Rappold HO. A comparative study between panoramic hysteroscopy with directed biopsies and dilatation and curettage. A review of 276 cases. Am J Obstet Gynecol 1988;158:489–92.
31. Loffer FD. Hysteroscopy with selective endometrial sampling compared with D&C for abnormal uterine bleeding: the value of a negative hysteroscopic view. Obstet Gynecol 1989;73:16–20.
32. Farquhar C, Ekeroma A, Furness S, et al. A systematic review of transvaginal ultrasonography, sonohysterography and hysteroscopy for the investigation of abnormal uterine bleeding in premenopausal women. Acta Obstet Gynecol Scand 2003;82:493–504.
33. Widrich T, Bradley LD, Mitchinson AR, et al. Comparison of saline infusion sonography with office hysteroscopy for the evaluation of the endometrium. Am J Obstet Gynecol 1996;174:1327–34.
34. Saidi MH, Sadler RK, Theis VD, et al. Comparison of sonography, sonohysterography, and hysteroscopy for evaluation of abnormal uterine bleeding. J Ultrasound Med 1997;16:587–91.
35. Munro MG, Brooks PG. Use of local anesthesia for office diagnostic and operative hysteroscopy. J Minim Invasive Gynecol 2010;17:709–18.
36. Dueholm M, Lundorf E, Hansen ES, et al. Evaluation of the uterine cavity with magnetic resonance imaging, transvaginal sonography, hysterosonographic examination, and diagnostic hysteroscopy. Fertil Steril 2001;76:350–7.
37. Dueholm M. Transvaginal ultrasound for diagnosis of adenomyosis: a review. Best Pract Res Clin Obstet Gynaecol 2006;20:569–82.
38. Chiang CH, Chang MY, Hsu JJ, et al. Tumor vascular pattern and blood flow impedance in the differential diagnosis of leiomyoma and adenomyosis by color Doppler sonography. J Assist Reprod Genet 1999;16:268–75.
39. Mark AS, Hricak H, Heinrichs LW, et al. Adenomyosis and leiomyoma: differential diagnosis with MR imaging. Radiology 1987;163:527–9.
40. Peddada SD, Laughlin SK, Miner K, et al. Growth of uterine leiomyomata among premenopausal black and white women. Proc Natl Acad Sci U S A 2008;105: 19887–92.
41. Tropeano G, Amoroso S, Scambia G. Non-surgical management of uterine fibroids. Hum Reprod Update 2008;14:259–74.

42. Lethaby A, Vollenhoven B, Sowter M. Pre-operative GnRH analogue therapy before hysterectomy or myomectomy for uterine fibroids. Cochrane Database Syst Rev 2001;2:CD000547.
43. Waibel-Treber S, Minne HW, Scharla SH, et al. Reversible bone loss in women treated with GnRH-agonists for endometriosis and uterine leiomyoma. Hum Reprod 1989;4:384–8.
44. Surrey ES, Hornstein MD. Prolonged GnRH agonist and add-back therapy for symptomatic endometriosis: long-term follow-up. Obstet Gynecol 2002;99:709–19.
45. Stovall TG, Muneyyirci-Delale O, Summitt RL Jr, et al. GnRH agonist and iron versus placebo and iron in the anemic patient before surgery for leiomyomas: a randomized controlled trial. Leuprolide Acetate Study Group. Obstet Gynecol 1995;86:65–71.
46. Benagiano G, Kivinen ST, Fadini R, et al. Zoladex (goserelin acetate) and the anemic patient: results of a multicenter fibroid study. Fertil Steril 1996;66:223–9.
47. Scialli AR, Jestila KJ. Sustained benefits of leuprolide acetate with or without subsequent medroxyprogesterone acetate in the nonsurgical management of leiomyomata uteri. Fertil Steril 1995;64:313–20.
48. Stovall TG, Ling FW, Henry LC, et al. A randomized trial evaluating leuprolide acetate before hysterectomy as treatment for leiomyomas. Am J Obstet Gynecol 1991;164: 1420–3 [discussion: 3–5].
49. Friedman AJ, Rein MS, Harrison-Atlas D, et al. A randomized, placebo-controlled, double-blind study evaluating leuprolide acetate depot treatment before myomectomy. Fertil Steril 1989;52:728–33.
50. Perino A, Chianchiano N, Petronio M, et al. Role of leuprolide acetate depot in hysteroscopic surgery: a controlled study. Fertil Steril 1993;59:507–10.
51. Phillips DR, Nathanson HG, Milim SJ, et al. The effect of dilute vasopressin solution on the force needed for cervical dilatation: a randomized controlled trial. Obstet Gynecol 1997;89:507–11.
52. Campo S, Campo V, Gambadauro P. Short-term and long-term results of resectoscopic myomectomy with and without pretreatment with GnRH analogs in premenopausal women. Acta Obstet Gynecol Scand 2005;84:756–60.
53. Mavrelos D, Ben-Nagi J, Davies A, et al. The value of pre-operative treatment with GnRH analogues in women with submucous fibroids: a double-blind, placebo-controlled randomized trial. Hum Reprod 2010;25:2264–9.
54. Muzii L, Boni T, Bellati F, et al. GnRH analogue treatment before hysteroscopic resection of submucous myomas: a prospective, randomized, multicenter study. Fertil Steril 2010;94:1496–9.
55. Soysal S, Soysal ME. The efficacy of levonorgestrel-releasing intrauterine device in selected cases of myoma-related menorrhagia: a prospective controlled trial. Gynecol Obstet Invest 2005;59:29–35.
56. Grigorieva V, Chen-Mok M, Tarasova M, et al. Use of a levonorgestrel-releasing intrauterine system to treat bleeding related to uterine leiomyomas. Fertil Steril 2003;79:1194–8.
57. Rein MS, Barbieri RL, Friedman AJ. Progesterone: a critical role in the pathogenesis of uterine myomas. Am J Obstet Gynecol 1995;172:14–8.
58. Rein MS. Advances in uterine leiomyoma research: the progesterone hypothesis. Environ Health Perspect 2000;108(Suppl 5):791–3.
59. Zhao K, Kuperman L, Geimonen E, et al. Progestin represses human connexin43 gene expression similarly in primary cultures of myometrial and uterine leiomyoma cells. Biol Reprod 1996;54:607–15.

60. Eisinger SH, Bonfiglio T, Fiscella K, et al. Twelve-month safety and efficacy of low-dose mifepristone for uterine myomas. J Minim Invasive Gynecol 2005;12: 227–33.
61. Carbonell Esteve JL, Acosta R, Heredia B, et al. Mifepristone for the treatment of uterine leiomyomas: a randomized controlled trial. Obstet Gynecol 2008;112: 1029–36.
62. Varelas FK, Papanicolaou AN, Vavatsi-Christaki N, et al. The effect of anastrazole on symptomatic uterine leiomyomata. Obstet Gynecol 2007;110:643–9.
63. Gurates B, Parmaksiz C, Kilic G, et al. Treatment of symptomatic uterine leiomyoma with letrozole. Reprod Biomed Online 2008;17:569–74.
64. Parsanezhad ME, Azmoon M, Alborzi S, et al. A randomized, controlled clinical trial comparing the effects of aromatase inhibitor (letrozole) and gonadotropin-releasing hormone agonist (triptorelin) on uterine leiomyoma volume and hormonal status. Fertil Steril 2009;93:192–8.
65. Atlee WL. Case of successful extirpation of a fibrous tumor of the peritoneal surface of the uterus by the large peritoneal section. Am J Med Sci 1845;9:309–35.
66. Bonney V. The technical minutia of extended myomectomy and ovarian cystectomy. London: Cassel; 1946.
67. Neuwirth RS. A new technique for and additional experience with hysteroscopic resection of submucous fibroids. Am J Obstet Gynecol 1978;131:91–4.
68. Semm K, Mettler L. Technical progress in pelvic surgery via operative laparoscopy. Am J Obstet Gynecol 1980;138:121–7.
69. Dubuisson JB, Lecuru F, Foulot H, et al Myomectomy by laparoscopy: a preliminary report of 43 cases. Fertil Steril 1991;56:827–30.
70. Fedele L, Vercellini P, Bianchi S, et al. Treatment with GnRH agonists before myomectomy and the risk of short-term myoma recurrence. Br J Obstet Gynaecol 1990;97:393–6.
71. Friedman AJ, Daly M, Juneau-Norcross M, et al. Recurrence of myomas after myomectomy in women pretreated with leuprolide acetate depot or placebo. Fertil Steril 1992;58:205–8.
72. Kongnyuy EJ, van den Broek N, Wiysonge CS. A systematic review of randomized controlled trials to reduce hemorrhage during myomectomy for uterine fibroids. Int J Gynaecol Obstet 2008;100:4–9.
73. Emanuel MH, Wamsteker K, Hart AA, et al. Long-term results of hysteroscopic myomectomy for abnormal uterine bleeding. Obstet Gynecol 1999;93:743–8.
74. Vercellini P, Zaina B, Yaylayan L, et al. Hysteroscopic myomectomy: long-term effects on menstrual pattern and fertility. Obstet Gynecol 1999;94:341–7.
75. Fernandez H, Sefrioui O, Virelizier C, et al. Hysteroscopic resection of submucosal myomas in patients with infertility. Hum Reprod 2001;16:1489–92.
76. Leone FP, Lanzani C, Ferrazzi E. Use of strict sonohysterographic methods for preoperative assessment of submucous myomas. Fertil Steril 2003;79:998–1002.
77. Propst AM, Liberman RF, Harlow BL, et al. Complications of hysteroscopic surgery: predicting patients at risk. Obstet Gynecol 2000;96:517–20.
78. Ginsburg ES, Benson CB, Garfield JM, et al. The effect of operative technique and uterine size on blood loss during myomectomy: a prospective randomized study. Fertil Steril 1993;60:956–62.
79. DeLancey JO. A modified technique for hemostasis during myomectomy. Surg Gynecol Obstet 1992;174:153–4.
80. Fletcher H, Frederick J, Hardie M, et al. A randomized comparison of vasopressin and tourniquet as hemostatic agents during myomectomy. Obstet Gynecol 1996; 87:1014–8.

81. Tulandi T, Murray C, Guralnick M. Adhesion formation and reproductive outcome after myomectomy and second-look laparoscopy. Obstet Gynecol 1993;82:213–5.

82. March CM, Boyers S, Franklin R, et al. Prevention of adhesion formation/reformation with the Gore-Tex Surgical Membrane. Prog Clin Biol Res 1993;381:253–9.

83. Mais V, Ajossa S, Piras B, et al. Prevention of de-novo adhesion formation after laparoscopic myomectomy: a randomized trial to evaluate the effectiveness of an oxidized regenerated cellulose absorbable barrier. Hum Reprod 1995;10:3133–5.

84. LaMorte AI, Lalwani S, Diamond MP. Morbidity associated with abdominal myomectomy. Obstet Gynecol 1993;82:897–900.

85. Nezhat FR, Roemisch M, Nezhat CH. Long-term follow-up of laparoscopic myomectomy. J Am Assoc Gynecol Laparosc 1996;3:S35.

86. Dubuisson JB, Chapron C, Verspyck E, et al. [Laparoscopic myomectomy. 102 cases]. Contracept Fertil Sex 1993;21:920–2 [in French].

87. Daniell JF, Kurtz BR, Taylor SN. Laparoscopic myomectomy using the argon beam coagulator. J Gynecol Surg 1993;9:207–12.

88. Parker WH, Rodi IA. Patient selection for laparoscopic myomectomy. J Am Assoc Gynecol Laparosc 1994;2:23–6.

89. Hasson HM, Rotman C, Rana N, et al. Laparoscopic myomectomy. Obstet Gynecol 1992;80:884–8.

90. Myers ER, Barber MD, Gustilo-Ashby T, et al. Management of uterine leiomyomata: what do we really know? Obstet Gynecol 2002;100:8–17.

91. Taylor A, Sharma M, Tsirkas P, et al. Reducing blood loss at open myomectomy using triple tourniquets: a randomised controlled trial. BJOG 2005;112:340–5.

92. Zullo F, Palomba S, Corea D, et al. Bupivacaine plus epinephrine for laparoscopic myomectomy: a randomized placebo-controlled trial. Obstet Gynecol 2004;104: 243–9.

93. Dubuisson JB, Fauconnier A, Deffarges JV, et al. Pregnancy outcome and deliveries following laparoscopic myomectomy. Hum Reprod 2000;15:869–73.

94. Mais V, Ajossa S, Guerriero S, et al. Laparoscopic versus abdominal myomectomy: a prospective, randomized trial to evaluate benefits in early outcome. Am J Obstet Gynecol 1996;174:654–8.

95. Carter JE, McCarus S. Time Savings Using the Steiner Morcellator in Laparoscopic Myomectomy. J Am Assoc Gynecol Laparosc 1996;3:S6.

96. Nezhat C, Nezhat F, Bess O, et al. Laparoscopically assisted myomectomy: a report of a new technique in 57 cases. Int J Fertil Menopausal Stud 1994;39:39–44.

97. Cagnacci A, Pirillo D, Malmusi S, et al. Early outcome of myomectomy by laparotomy, minilaparotomy and laparoscopically assisted minilaparotomy. A randomized prospective study. Hum Reprod 2003;18:2590–4.

98. Goldrath MH. Vaginal removal of the pedunculated submucous myoma: the use of laminaria. Obstet Gynecol 1987;70:670–2.

99. Goldrath MH. Vaginal removal of the pedunculated submucous myoma. Historical observations and development of a new procedure. J Reprod Med 1990;35:921–4.

100. Ravina JH, Merland JJ, Ciraru-Vigneron N, et al. [Arterial embolization: a new treatment of menorrhagia in uterine fibroma]. Presse Med 1995;24:1754 [in French].

101. Pinto I, Chimeno P, Romo A, et al. Uterine fibroids: uterine artery embolization versus abdominal hysterectomy for treatment–a prospective, randomized, and controlled clinical trial. Radiology 2003;226:425–31.

102. Hehenkamp WJ, Volkers NA, Donderwinkel PF, et al. Uterine artery embolization versus hysterectomy in the treatment of symptomatic uterine fibroids (EMMY trial): peri- and postprocedural results from a randomized controlled trial. Am J Obstet Gynecol 2005;193:1618–29.

103. Spies JB, Ascher SA, Roth AR, et al. Uterine artery embolization for leiomyomata. Obstet Gynecol 2001;98:29–34.

104. Spies JB, Bruno J, Czeyda-Pommersheim F, et al. Long-term outcome of uterine artery embolization of leiomyomata. Obstet Gynecol 2005;106:933–9.

105. Goodwin SC, Spies JB, Worthington-Kirsch R, et al. Uterine artery embolization for treatment of leiomyomata: long-term outcomes from the FIBROID Registry. Obstet Gynecol 2008;111:22–33.

106. Coleman P. Systematic review of the efficacy and safety of uterine artery embolisation in the treatment of fibroids. London: National Institute for Clinical Excellence; 2004.

107. Gupta JK, Sinha AS, Lumsden MA, et al. Uterine artery embolization for symptomatic uterine fibroids. Cochrane Database Syst Rev 2006;1:CD005073.

108. Pron G, Mocarski E, Bennett J, et al. Pregnancy after uterine artery embolization for leiomyomata: the Ontario multicenter trial. Obstet Gynecol 2005;105:67–76.

109. Carpenter TT, Walker WJ. Pregnancy following uterine artery embolisation for symptomatic fibroids: a series of 26 completed pregnancies. BJOG 2005;112: 321–5.

110. Pinto Pabon I, Magret JP, Unzurrunzaga EA, et al. Pregnancy after uterine fibroid embolization: follow-up of 100 patients embolized using tris-acryl gelatin microspheres. Fertil Steril 2008;90:2356–60.

111. Agdi M, Valenti D, Tulandi T. Intraabdominal adhesions after uterine artery embolization. American J Obstet Gynecol 2008;199:482 e1–3.

112. Liu WM, Ng HT, Wu YC, et al. Laparoscopic bipolar coagulation of uterine vessels: a new method for treating symptomatic fibroids. Fertil Steril 2001;75:417–22.

113. Lichtinger M, Hallson L, Calvo P, et al. Laparoscopic uterine artery occlusion for symptomatic leiomyomas. J Am Assoc Gynecol Laparosc 2002;9:191–8.

114. Park KH, Kim JY, Shin JS, et al. Treatment outcomes of uterine artery embolization and laparoscopic uterine artery ligation for uterine myoma. Yonsei Med J 2003;44: 694–702.

115. Hald K, Klow NE, Qvigstad E, et al. Laparoscopic occlusion compared with embolization of uterine vessels: a randomized controlled trial. Obstet Gynecol 2007;109: 20–7.

116. Cunningham E, Barreda L, Ngo M, et al. Uterine artery embolization versus occlusion for uterine leiomyomas: a pilot randomized clinical trial. J Minim Invasive Gynecol 2008;15:301–7.

117. Farquhar CM, Steiner CA. Hysterectomy rates in the United States 1990–1997. Obstet Gynecol 2002;99:229–34.

118. Olive DL, Rutherford T, Zreik T, et al. Cryomyolysis in the conservative treatment of uterine fibroids. J Am Assoc Gynecol Laparosc 1996;3:S36.

119. Devireddy RV, Coad JE, Bischof JC. Microscopic and calorimetric assessment of freezing processes in uterine fibroid tumor tissue. Cryobiology 2001;42:225–43.

120. Rupp CC, Nagel TC, Swanlund DJ, et al. Cryothermic and hyperthermic treatments of human leiomyomata and adjacent myometrium and their implications for laparoscopic surgery. J Am Assoc Gynecol Laparosc 2003;10:90–8.

121. Zreik TG, Rutherford TJ, Palter SF, et al. Cryomyolysis, a new procedure for the conservative treatment of uterine fibroids. J Am Assoc Gynecol Laparosc 1998;5: 33–8.

122. Odnusi KO, Rutherford TJ, Olive DL, et al. Cryomyolysis in the management of uterine fibroids: technique and complications. Surg Technol Int 2000;8:173–8.

123. Zupi E, Piredda A, Marconi D, et al. Directed laparoscopic cryomyolysis: a possible alternative to myomectomy and/or hysterectomy for symptomatic leiomyomas. Am J Obstet Gynecol 2004;190:639–43.

124. Ciavattini A, Tsiroglou D, Piccioni M, et al. Laparoscopic cryomyolysis: an alternative to myomectomy in women with symptomatic fibroids. Surg Endosc 2004;18:1785–8.

125. Zupi E, Marconi D, Sbracia M, et al. Directed laparoscopic cryomyolysis for symptomatic leiomyomata: one-year follow up. J Minim Invasive Gynecol 2005;12:343–6.

126. Ciavattini A, Tsiroglou D, Litta P, et al. Pregnancy outcome after laparoscopic cryomyolysis of uterine myomas: report of nine cases. J Minim Invasive Gynecol 2006;13:141–4.

127. Nisolle M, Smets M, Malvaux V, et al. Laparoscopic myolysis with the Nd:YAG laser. J Gynecol Surg 1993;9:95–9.

128. Zaporozhan VN. Intratissue laser thermotherapy in treatment of uterine myomata. J Am Assoc Gynecol Laparosc 1996;3:S56.

129. Jourdain O, Roux D, Cambon D, et al. A new method for the treatment of fibromas: interstitial laser hyperthermia using the Nd:YAG laser. Preliminary study. Eur J Obstet Gynecol Reprod Biol 1996;64:73–8.

130. Goldfarb HA. Comparison of bipolar electrocoagulation and Nd:YAG laser coagulation for symptomatic reduction of uterine myomas. J Am Assoc Gynecol Laparosc 1994;1:S13.

131. Phillips DR, Milim SJ, Nathanson HG, et al. Experience with laparoscopic leiomyoma coagulation and concomitant operative hysteroscopy. J Am Assoc Gynecol Laparosc 1997;4:425–33.

132. Hurst BS, Elliot M, Matthews ML, et al. Ultrasound-directed transvaginal myolysis: preclinical studies. J Minim Invasive Gynecol 2007;14:502–5.

133. Arcangeli S, Pasquarette MM. Gravid uterine rupture after myolysis. Obstet Gynecol 1997;89:857.

134. Vilos GA, Daly LJ, Tse BM. Pregnancy outcome after laparoscopic electromyolysis. J Am Assoc Gynecol Laparosc 1998;5:289–92.

135. Tempany CM, Stewart EA, McDannold N, et al. MR imaging-guided focused ultrasound surgery of uterine leiomyomas: a feasibility study. Radiology 2003;226:897–905.

136. Lynn JG, Zwerner, RL, Chick, AJ, et al. A new method for the generation and use of focused ultrasound in experimental biology. J Gen Physiol 1942;26:179–203.

137. Hynynen K, Pomeroy O, Smith DN, et al. MR imaging-guided focused ultrasound surgery of fibroadenomas in the breast: a feasibility study. Radiology 2001;219:176–85.

138. McDannold N, Moss M, Killiany R, et al. MRI-guided focused ultrasound surgery in the brain: tests in a primate model. Magn Reson Med 2003;49:1188–91.

139. Smith NB, Buchanan MT, Hynynen K. Transrectal ultrasound applicator for prostate heating monitored using MRI thermometry. Int J Radiat Oncol Biol Phys 1999;43:217–25.

140. Zhou XD, Ren XL, Zhang J, et al. Therapeutic response assessment of high intensity focused ultrasound therapy for uterine fibroid: utility of contrast-enhanced ultrasonography. Eur J Radiol 2007;62:289–94.

141. Hynynen K, Freund WR, Cline HE, et al. A clinical, noninvasive, MR imaging-monitored ultrasound surgery method. Radiographics 1996;16:185–95.

142. Chung AH, Jolesz FA, Hynynen K. Thermal dosimetry of a focused ultrasound beam in vivo by magnetic resonance imaging. Med Phys 1999;26:2017–26.

143. Stewart EA, Gedroyc WM, Tempany CM, et al. Focused ultrasound treatment of uterine fibroid tumors: safety and feasibility of a noninvasive thermoablative technique. Am J Obstet Gynecol 2003;189:48–54.
144. Hindley J, Gedroyc WM, Regan L, et al. MRI guidance of focused ultrasound therapy of uterine fibroids: early results. AJR Am J Roentgenol 2004;183:1713–9.
145. Stewart EA, Rabinovici J, Tempany CM, et al. Clinical outcomes of focused ultrasound surgery for the treatment of uterine fibroids. Fertil Steril 2006;85:22–9.
146. Smart OC, Hindley JT, Regan L, et al. Gonadotrophin-releasing hormone and magnetic-resonance-guided ultrasound surgery for uterine leiomyomata. Obstet Gynecol 2006;108:49–54.
147. Smart OC, Hindley JT, Regan L, et al. Magnetic resonance guided focused ultrasound surgery of uterine fibroids–the tissue effects of GnRH agonist pre-treatment. Eur J Radiol 2006;59:163–7.
148. McDannold N, Tempany CM, Fennessy FM, et al. Uterine leiomyomas: MR imaging-based thermometry and thermal dosimetry during focused ultrasound thermal ablation. Radiology 2006;240:263–72.

Simulation and Education in Gynecologic Surgery

Marshall L. Smith, MD, PhD[a,b,c],*

KEYWORDS

• Simulation • Surgery • Training • Education
• Error reduction

Simulation training has suddenly become the rage in healthcare, with every week some new center marketing themselves as the first simulation training center in the area. Most announcements elaborate upon the attributes of this "brand new" technology, when in fact most other industries have used sophisticated simulation training for decades . . . and healthcare is only now trying to catch up! Aviation and nuclear energy are only 2 of the many industries that have for years embedded simulation into both their education and quality improvement programs. Aviation is noteworthy in that today a regularly scheduled assessment on sophisticated flight simulators is a well-ingrained part of an airline pilot's maintenance of licensure and accreditation. As in gynecologic surgery today, the simulators in aviation also started with very simple models when Edwin Link developed the first flight simulator in 1929, the precursor of the modern-day flight simulator.[1] Today's flight simulators are sophisticated virtual reality trainers that can be used not only to train, but to evaluate, a pilot's skills under all possible conditions and malfunctions. Aviation's crew resource management program is the other component of their flight crew training in which simulation training is used to develop proficient levels of communication, leadership and team dynamics, namely, team training. These principles have also been used to develop team training programs for use in healthcare, as with such programs as TeamSTEPPS which was developed jointly by the Agency for Healthcare Research and Quality and the United States Department of Defense Patient Safety Program.[2] This type of team training and simulation is becoming increasingly recognized as another necessary component to help reduce errors in surgery today; and although simulation is beginning to be used for operating room (OR) teams and surgeons, those discussions are beyond the scope of this article.

The author has nothing to disclose.
[a] SimET Center Banner Good Samaritan Medical Center, WT-1, 1111 East McDowell Road, Phoenix, AZ 85006, USA
[b] Department of Obstetrics & Gynecology, University of Arizona, Tucson, AZ, USA
[c] Biomedical Informatics, Arizona State University, Phoenix, AZ, USA
* Corresponding author. Clinical Education and Innovation, Banner Health, Banner Good Samaritan Medical Center, WT-1, 1111 East McDowell Road, Phoenix, AZ 85006.
E-mail address: Mark.Smith@Bannerhealth.com

Obstet Gynecol Clin N Am 38 (2011) 733–740
doi:10.1016/j.ogc.2011.09.007
0889-8545/11/$ – see front matter © 2011 Elsevier Inc. All rights reserved.

Simulation training in surgery is not even novel in healthcare; in 800 BC Sushruta (the father of surgery) recommended the practice on melons and wormed wood for training for his students for surgery.[3] The well-recognized apprentice method of training (see one, do one, teach one) was developed over 3000 years ago in ancient Greece, and yet after all these centuries it continues to be the default method of surgical training. Additionally, this technique has remained essentially unchanged over this time despite being employed in an industry that is caring for sicker and sicker patients treated with increasingly complicated procedures. Fortunately, this method of teaching is finally becoming recognized to be outdated, inefficient, and dangerous in today's complex surgical environments. This recognition coupled with a growing awareness and impatience with high error rates in healthcare is driving a mandate that alternative and safer methods of training be developed and implemented, and simulation has emerged as one of leading solutions and answers to this challenge.

David Gaba, considered by many as the father of simulation training, introduced the modern era of simulation in healthcare when he introduced and promoted mannequin training in the late 1980s.[4] Thus, anesthesia has been using simulation training with mannequins for years, and only within the last decade has the field of surgery begun to recognize the value and embrace the concept of surgical simulation. There were other early pioneers in surgical education who also advocated moving away from the traditional apprentice method and to the incorporation of more objective measures for surgical training. Nearly 20 years ago, Reznik called for moving away from the subjective approach of visually assessing a trainee's skills and employing more objective metrics,[5] and Darzi and colleagues[6] argued in 1999 that more objectivity is needed in surgical training and assessment. One of the early visionaries in gynecology, Goff and associates[7] recommended a more formal and objective approach to the teaching of surgical skills. And even as early as 1993, Satava[8] published a prediction that virtual reality simulators would be the next big step in surgical training. During this time period, it also began to be recognized and documented that practice outside of the OR (in a simulated environment using either box trainers or virtual reality) was more effective than traditional methods for developing operative skills.[9-11] This growing awareness of the value of simulation was developing about the same time of the publication of the Institute of Medicine's (IOM) landmark publication *To Err is Human*, which first exposed to the public the high error rates in healthcare in 1999,[12] and follow-up reports only continued to confirm the same problem. Two years later, the IOM published a second report *Crossing the Quality Chasm,*[13] which stated that "The present system cannot do the job! Trying harder will not work. Changing systems of care will!" This second report advocated the adoption of simulation training as a possible solution to the high error rates in healthcare. The ensuing transition and integration of simulation into surgical educa-tion in the first part of this decade was reviewed in an excellent overview in this series by Chou and Handa in 2006.[14]

ATTRIBUTES AND COMPONENTS OF SIMULATION

There are a wide variety of surgical simulators available today, all with varying levels of sophistication. They are often classified as either high or low fidelity, which implies differing levels of realism relative to the actual task. That said, a simulator should be used to help develop or acquire a specific skill, and should be matched to both the needs of the training (including cost considerations) as well as the learning objectives. Box trainers may be of lower fidelity than virtual reality simulators but certainly continue to provide value in training, and the Foundations of Laparoscopic Surgery is a perfect example.[15] Likewise, more electronically sophisticated simulators can often meet more specific training needs and objectives, which should always be the primary objective for the adoption of simulation or simulators. Virtual reality simulators may also have learning modules imbedded in them, often eliminating the need for an instructor when practicing and learning. Simulators have to be validated to ensure that they are teaching the intended skills, that they can differentiate between different levels of those skills, and that their results are reproducible. It is critical when teaching surgical skills that a simulator (of any kind) is able to differentiate between learners with different levels of skills to determine whether there is any progress in learning or skill acquisition. This is termed construct validity, and is only one of the several important levels of validation. Consistently showing the same measurements from the same skill levels is also important if one wants to rely on the results (reliability). And predictive validity and transference (do the acquired skills transfer to the actual OR) are obviously the ultimate criteria of a simulator's value.

Simulation training does bring new capabilities to teaching over more traditional methods. Simulation learning allows the learner the "ability to practice and learn in a consequence-free environment." Over the years, essentially all surgeons have learned their surgical skills while operating on their or their attending's patients. However, on a live patient a trainee usually has only 1 attempt to get it right, and then the patient (and the surgeon) must live with that result. This is a very slow, and often dangerous, way to learn . . . being overly cautious so as not to cause any harm to the patient. And, no one would ever suggest that a trainee should go into surgery and practice a procedure over and over on a live patient. Herein lies the value of simulation learning; surgeons can practice a task or skill over and over until it is learned and committed to automation, and there are no serious consequences if a mistake is made in practice on inanimate simulators.

The other landmark quality of simulation training is that finally one has the ability to quantitatively measure skill levels. Simulation allows the use of standardized exercises where the identical exercise can be performed over and over, with objective computerized metrics of progress when improving one's skill levels. In the past, evaluation of surgeons' skills have been relegated to either subjective or simple objective assessments by expert faculty surgeons, who would in turn then subjectively state when a surgeon was ready to move on to the next level or year of training, and often not because of any particular objective data but because they felt they could tell a good surgeon when they saw one. Even afterward, when surgeons started practice and applied for privileges at their hospital, they would often be supervised by a biased peer, who watched them in surgery and then declared them to be competent surgically as long as there were no major complications. Efforts are underway today to improve the interrater reliability of surgical auditors by the American College of Surgeons' NSQIP program, and great strides have been made in reducing variations between observers.[16,17] However, the variations in the countless presentations of actual surgical patients with varying diagnoses and levels of severity still make benchmarking in the live OR extremely difficult.

In the early part of the last decade, surgical and gynecologic residencies all began to integrate simulation and virtual reality training into their curricula and learning programs. During this early adoption phase of simulation with more objectivity increasingly being applied to training and assessment, the next question to answer was how well skills acquired in simulation training, of any type, were then carried into the OR when operating on a live patient. This is called transference, and there is now a significant amount of evidence that shows that proper simulation training with focused practice does develop technical surgical skills that transfer into the OR on live patients.[15,18-22] Simulation and simulators continue to bring even more value into the assessments of surgical skills, and will be a valuable tool in the future for both training and evaluating a surgeon's skill levels.

A TIME OF TRANSITION

The American College of Surgeons has led all the other surgical specialties in this adoption of simulation as a learning tool, and general surgery was the first surgical specialty to mandate that simulation would be a part of every accredited Residency in General Surgery.[23] In 2007, the American College of Surgeons endorsed the Foundations of Laparoscopic Surgery, a web-based program that also includes a box trainer for the assessment of manual skills. This is a joint venture between the American College of Surgeons and The Society of American Gastrointestinal and Endoscopic Surgeons; today, the successful completion of this module is a prerequisite for sitting for the boards in general surgery.[24] The American Board of Obstetrics and Gynecology, the American Congress of Obstetricians and Gynecologists, and the American Association of Gynecologic Laparoscopists are also seeking a similar gynecologic surgical simulator to train and evaluate resident learning of surgical skills in gynecology (personal communication from speakers at Medicine Meets Virtual Reality annual meeting, 2011).

Simbionix, CAE, Surgical Science, METI, and Mentice are a few of the many companies offering surgical simulators today, with newer technology appearing rapidly, and this has helped to drive awareness of simulation in the field of gynecology. What seemed to be the "critical mass" over the last decade was the approval of carotid stenting by the US Food and Drug Administration in 2004, but limited only for physicians who had first been trained by simulation.[25] This was the first time the US Food and Drug Administration had ever commented or required any type of training, and many educators thought this was the stimulus that was going to catapult simulation training into the mainstream, and indeed it probably did help.

But likely even more important as a stimulus, education in healthcare has been becoming under increasingly scrutiny for years as to its adequacy for training healthcare providers for today's increased complexity of caring for and operating upon patients. On the 10th anniversary of *To Err is Human*, the IOM yet again published a revealing but disheartening commentary (*Redesigning Continuing Education in the Health Professions*) on the status of continuing education and training in healthcare in the United States today by describing it as "woefully inadequate."[26] Other factors also appeared during these times that too are driving the adoption of simulation training. Reduced resident work hours, decreasing numbers of patients and thus learning cases, and increasing pressure from regulatory agencies and credentialing organizations, third-party reimbursement companies, and the general public are all drivers pressuring to make surgical training more efficient and thus reduce errors and complications; that is, finding a better way of training and measuring surgeons' skills.

It also has been long recognized that a good surgeon possess more than just technical skills, and that there are many other qualities that contribute to a surgeon's competence. In the last few years, more attention has been directed to the cognitive components of surgeons' skills and how to train and assess them, and some researchers such as Kahol and associates have begun to integrate measures of cognitive skills into simulators.[27] Every gynecologic faculty knows that critical thinking skills are absolutely essential to become a good surgeon, but all residency directors and faculty educators strain to find a way to even define them, much less train for and measure them. And, even when psychomotor and cognitive skills are objectively measured in a surgeon, they can be significantly altered by environmental factors such as an improvement with warming up before starting the surgery[28] or a significant degradation of (especially cognitive) skills with fatigue after a night of being on call.[29] Other qualities of a competent surgeon certainly include a vast knowledge and experiential base, along with the cognitive skills that seem to develop with experience in most surgeons. Supporters of the use of simulation in surgery often mention the aviation industry with its flight simulators, where very sophisticated virtual experiences and assessments that have contributed to one of the lowest error rates of any industry in the world. But whereas aviation has fully embraced simulation training both for pilot's skills as well as for teamwork training, even there it is not the final test! And when resident surgeons in training have fully automated their surgical skills with simulators and simulation, there will always be a need for a proctor standing by when the trainee standing over his or her patient first calls for a scalpel, just as there will always be flight proctors in the aviation industry when a new pilot first takes the throttle.

THE FUTURE OF SIMULATION IN SURGERY

The winds of change are certainly beginning to blow for more increased accountability in healthcare, and closely behind that will be ongoing surgical assessments for skill levels throughout a surgeon's professional career. Nearly all stakeholders in healthcare agree that these coming changes will be transformative. As mentioned, these growing demands for reduction of errors and improvement of quality in all healthcare areas certainly include the surgical arena, and accompanying these changes is a sense of growing importance of simulation as a more efficient training and assessment tool over the traditional subjective assessments of centuries past. The IOM's *Redesigning Continuing Education in the Health Professions* in 2010 focused on the status of healthcare in the area of education not only for residents but for all gynecologic surgeons in reference to lifelong learning.[26] Quotes from this article include:

- "Today in the United States, the professional health workforce is not consistently prepared to provide high quality health care and assure patient safety."
- "The absence of a comprehensive and well-integrated system of continuing education . . . in the health professions is an important contributing factor to knowledge and performance deficiencies at the individual and system levels."

Programs addressing these improved training and assessment needs will certainly include simulation as a resource to meet these ongoing educational requirements in gynecologic surgery, not only for surgical skill evaluations, but also for learning how to safely perform new procedures and use new medical devices as they continually evolve in the OR.

The introduction and growth of minimally invasive surgery also facilitates the integration of simulation into surgical assessment and training; there is now a digital signal and record of each surgery. The movements of both the instruments as well as those of the surgeon's hands during the performance of a simulation procedure or exercise can now be recorded digitally and correlated with the results and outcomes of the provided exercises in training.[26] This technique will eventually provide instructors and evaluators with objective data to more objectively assess skill levels. The problem at the time of the writing of this article is that the methodology has not yet been sufficiently developed to accomplish the required granularity of assessments on this data; however, but most recognized experts agree that this will be the means with which the best objectivity will be applied to the evaluation of surgeons' skills, especially in the field of minimally invasive surgery.

All these factors present several challenges in surgical training and assessment that await us. First, all of the components of competency will have to be more clearly defined, and a set of objective metrics developed for measuring those competencies. This methodology will have to include assessment of both the cognitive and critical thinking elements. Second, these metrics will need to be standardized, so that when a gynecologic surgeon's skills are measured for ABOG credentialing the metrics obtained in New England will mean the same as those obtained on the West Coast. Third, there will need to be a national database of skill levels, so that benchmarking of skill levels can occur. This is something most surgeons prefer not to hear, but the consensus is rapidly growing that if it is not done from within the specialty, then it will be mandated from the outside by nonphysician regulatory agencies. This oncoming challenge is not going away and is rapidly becoming obstetrician/gynecologist's own burning platform.

The question many ask is what form simulation will take into the future as it is increasingly included as a resource to meet the changing needs in surgery. Certainly a more standardized, objective, and reliable methodology of assessing surgeons' skills and competencies, at all levels of training and with continued assessment throughout their professional career, will be required. Simulation will be employed to both train and assess cognitive and critical thinking skills in addition to other critical components of surgeons' overall competency as those other contributory factors become more clearly defined. These metrics will likely be increasingly employed for maintenance of specialty credentialing in obstetrics and gynecology and for mainte-nance of state licensure. These measurements will be used for privileging of physicians for hospitals, and for Ongoing Provider Professional Evaluation, an ongoing monitoring of physicians skill levels recently mandated by the joint commis-sion. Instead of consisting of reactive oversight with a punitive purpose, ongoing assessments in simulation should be used to detect early degradation of surgical skills, so that a surgeon can be remediated or his/her practice redirected instead of allowing the physician to get into serious trouble in the OR by making errors, or even worse, causing an injury or death.

CONCLUSION

In the surgical world we live in today, where new procedures, drugs, medical devices, and operative protocols are constantly being developed, and then quickly altered again, practitioners must have ongoing programs of self-learning and assessment if they are to remain current and provide the best care possible to those that depend upon and trust them—their patients. Different forms of simulation learning will continue to evolve to provide surgeons one of the educational modalities to provide that support in today's busy and increasingly complex practice of gynecologic surgery.

ACKNOWLEDGMENT

The author acknowledges his colleague Kanav Kahol, PhD, for support for this article.

REFERENCES

1. Helleberg JR, Wickens CD. Effects of data-link modality and display redundancy on pilot performance: an attentional perspective. The International Journal of Aviation Psychology 2003;13:189–210.
2. Clancy CM, Tornberg DM. TeamSTEPPS: assuring optimal teamwork in clinical settings. Am J Med Qual 2007;22:214–6.

3. Saraf S, Parihar RS. Sushruta: the first plastic surgeon in 600 B.C. The Internet Journal of Plastic Surgery 2007:4:2.
4. Rosen KR. The history of medical simulation. J Crit Care 2008;23:157–66.
5. Reznick RK. Teaching and testing technical skills. Am J Surg 1993;3:358–61.
6. Darzi A, Smith S, Taffinder N. Assessing operative skill needs to become more objective. BMJ 1999;318:887.
7. Goff BA, Lentz GM, Lee DM, et al. Formal teaching of surgical skills in an obstetric-gynecologic residency. Obstet Gynecol 1999;93:785–90.
8. Satava RM. Virtual reality surgical simulator. Surg Endosc 1993;7:203–5.
9. Rosser JC, Rosser LE, Savalgi RS. Skill acquisition and assessment for laparoscopic surgery. Arch Surg 1997;132:200–4.
10. Scott DJ, Bergen PC, Rege RV, et al. Laparoscopic training on bench models: better and more cost effective than operating room experience? J Am Coll Surg 2000;191: 272–83.
11. Hyltander A, Liljegren E, Rhodin PH, et al. The transfer of basic skills learned in a laparoscopic simulator to the operating room. Surg Endosc 2002;16:1324–8.
12. US Institute of Medicine. Committee on Quality of Health. To err is human: building a safer health system. Washington, DC: National Academy Press; 1999.
13. US Institute of Medicine. Committee on Quality of Health Care in America. Crossing the quality chasm: a new health system for the 21st century. Washington, DC: National Academy Press; 2001.
14. Chou B, Handa VL. Simulators and virtual reality in surgical education. Obstet Gynecol Clin North Am 2006;33:283–96.
15. McCluney AL, Vassiliou MC, Kaneva PA, et al. FLS Simulator performance predicts intraoperative laparoscopic skill. Surg Endosc 2007;21:1991–5.
16. Van Hove PD, Tuijthof GJM, Verdaasdonk EGG, et al. Objective assessment of technical surgical skills. Br J Surg 2010;97:972–87.
17. Mira Shiloach M, Frencher SK Jr, Steeger JE, et al. Toward robust information: data quality and inter-rater reliability in the American College of Surgeons National Surgical Quality Improvement Program. J Am Coll Surg 2010;210:6–16.
18. Seymour NE, Gallagher AG, Roman SA, et al. Virtual reality training improves operating room performance: results of a randomized, double-blinded study. Ann Surg 2002;236:458–63.
19. Grantcharov TP, Kristiansen VB, Bendix J, et al. Randomized clinical trial of virtual reality simulation for laparoscopic skills training. Br J Surg 2004;91:146–50.
20. Munz Y, Kumar BD, Moorthy K, et al. Laparoscopic virtual reality and box trainers: is one superior to the other? Surg Endosc 2004;18:485–94.
21. Sturm LP, Windsor JA, Cosman PH, et al. A systematic review of skills transfer after surgical simulation training. Ann Surg 2008;248:166–79.
22. Gurusamy K, Aggarwal R, Palanivelu L, et al. Systematic review of randomized controlled trials on the effectiveness of virtual reality training for laparoscopic surgery. J Surg 2008;95:1088–97.
23. Sachdeva AK, Pelligrini CA, Johnson KA. Support for simulation-based surgical education through American College of Surgeons Accredited Education Institutes. World J Surg 2008;32:196–207.
24. Sroka G, Feldman LS, Vassiliou MC, et al. Fundamentals of Laparoscopic Surgery simulator training to proficiency improves laparoscopic performance in the operating room—a randomized controlled trial. Am J Surg 2010;199:115–20.
25. Gallagher A, Cates C. Approval of virtual reality training for carotid stenting: what this means for procedural-based medicine. JAMA 2004;292:3024–6.

26. Institute of Medicine, Committee on Planning a Continuing Health Care Professional Education Institute. Redesigning continuing education in the health professions. Washington, DC: National Academy Press; 2010. Available at: http://www.nap.edu/openbook.php?record_id=12704. Accessed September 21, 2011.

27. Kahol K, Vankipuram M, Smith ML. Cognitive simulators for medical education and training. J Biomed Informatics 2009;42:593–604.

28. Kahol K, Satava RM, Ferrara J, et al. Effect of short-term pretrial practice on surgical proficiency in simulated environments: a randomized trial of the "preoperative warm-up" effect. J Am Coll Surg 2009;208:255–68.

29. Kahol K, Leyba MJ, Deka M, et al. Effect of fatigue on psychomotor and cognitive skills. Am J Surg 2008;195:195–204.

Laparoendoscopic Single-Site Surgery in Gynecology

Craig Sobolewski, MD[a],*, Patrick P. Yeung Jr, MD[b],
Stuart Hart, MD[c]

KEYWORDS

- Gynecologic procedures
- Laparo-endoscopic single-site surgery
- Minimally invasive surgery • Technology

Laparoscopic surgery has become the standard approach for many gynecologic procedures. The benefits of this approach over laparotomy relating to recovery, decreased morbidity, quality of life, and cosmesis are well established.[1-3] In the last decade, there have been multiple advances in the technology of minimally invasive surgery enabling more complex procedures to be offered via a less invasive approach. Examples include advanced imaging platforms such as digital cameras and high definition monitors, suture-assist devices, "smart" energy devices, and robotics.

Traditional operative laparoscopic surgery is performed via a multiport approach. This allows for the creation of triangulation to the target organ or tissue. Requisite to this approach is the placement of ports lateral to midline. Placement in these locations can be a source of potential morbidity. Injury to the inferior epigastric vessels has been reported to be the most common complication in laparoscopically assisted vaginal hysterectomy (LAVH) with an incidence of 24 per 1000 cases.[4] Lateral ports may be a source of significant neuropathic pain if the iliohypogastric or ilioinguinal nerves are injured during the placement of the trocars or the repair of the incision site. After operative laparoscopy, hernias at the site of the laparoscopic port are more likely to occur in the lateral accessory ports than at the umbilicus.[5]

Although not a new concept, the idea of performing minimally invasive operative procedures through a single incision, thus eliminating the potential risk associated

Disclosures: Craig Sobolewski serves as a consultant and speaker for Covidien, Inc, a consultant for TransEnterix, and on the advisory board of CareFusion. Patrick P. Yeung serves as a consultant and speaker for Covidien, Inc. Stuart Hart serves as a consultant and speaker for Covidien, Inc.
[a] Duke University Medical Center, 3116 North Duke Street, Durham, NC 27704, USA
[b] Saint Louis University, St. Louis, MO, USA
[c] University of South Florida, 2 Tampa General Circle, 4th Floor, Tampa, FL 33606, USA
* Corresponding author.
E-mail address:craig.sobolewski@duke.edu

with lateral assistant ports, has recently enjoyed a renewed interest. Significant advances in technology have helped to foster much of this interest.

It should be noted that a single puncture approach to access the peritoneal cavity has been described utilizing a variety of names. One of the earliest terms, single-port access surgery, was trademarked by Drexel University.[6] In part because of a lack of uniformity in terminology and the implications this could have on searching for evidence-based reports on this technique, a panel of experts was recently assembled as the Laparoendoscopic Single Site Consortium for Assessment and Research to address this and similar issues. This group has suggested that the term laparoendoscopic single-site surgery (LESS) best encompasses this approach across all specialties and has encouraged its use in scientific publications.[7]

HISTORICAL PERSPECTIVES
Gynecology

A single-puncture approach for the performance of relatively straightforward procedures has been utilized in gynecologic surgery for decades. Using an offset operative laparoscope, Wheeless[8] first described the advantages of a single puncture approach for the performance of laparoscopic sterilizations in 1969. He went on to describe the safety of this approach in a series of more than 3000 patients.[9] Pelosi and Pelosi[10] described the first report of a single-puncture laparoscopic hysterectomy in 1991, again utilizing an offset operative laparoscope to perform the procedure. Despite several additional publications demonstrating its feasibility, this approach was never popularized until recent technology developments have spawned a renewed interest in this approach.[11-14] Reports of a single-puncture approach for a variety of gynecologic procedures, including adnexal procedures and hysterectomy, did not appear again in the published medical literature until this decade.

General Surgery

The first LESS cholecystectomy was performed by Navarra and colleagues in 1997.[15] They utilized 1 skin incision through which they placed two, 10-mm trocars. Retraction of the gallbladder was accomplished via 3 sutures placed into it through the abdominal wall. Since that first report, there have been at least 35 published series on LESS cholecystectomy.[6] Espisito reported on the first single incision laparoscopic appendectomy in 1998.[6]

Urology

Hirono and colleagues reported on the first LESS experience in urologic surgery in 2005.[16] They utilized a 4-cm resectoscope tube to perform retroperitoneoscopic adrenalectomy without insufflation. Other LESS urologic procedures include pyeloplasty, nephrectomy and prostatectomy.[6] Innovation and creativity are common denominators in the early experiences with LESS procedures.

LESS INSTRUMENTATION

The performance of a LESS hysterectomy procedure requires instrumentation that enables the surgeon to compensate for the many challenges encountered during single-port surgery. Loss of triangulation, instrument collision/sword fighting, and difficulty with tissue manipulation are especially problematic during these operative procedures. Fortunately, instrumentation is available to allow surgeons to overcome many of these challenges.

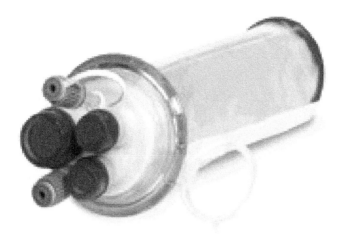

Fig. 1. Triport (*Courtesy of* Olympus America, Inc, Center Valley, PA; with permission.).

Uterine Manipulation

Effective uterine manipulation is essential during a LESS hysterectomy procedure. In a traditional, multiport, total laparoscopic hysterectomy (TLH) procedure, the uterus can be efficiently manipulated using laparoscopic instruments through any auxiliary port. During a LESS hysterectomy procedure, the surgeon has a limited ability to manipulate the uterus in this manner, and the use of a uterine manipulator' can essentially act as an additional port to efficiently manipulate the uterus. This enables the surgeon full uterine manipulation without the inherent mobility limitations imposed by the use of a single-incision port. The more common uterine manipulators currently available include the RUMI uterine manipulator with KOH colpotomizer (Cooper Surgical, Trumbull, CT, USA), Pelosi uterine manipulator (Apple Medical Corporation, Marlborough, MA, USA), and the VCare uterine manipulator (ConMed Corporation, Utica, NY, USA).

Each uterine manipulator has unique advantages and disadvantages. The RUMI Uterine Manipulator has 140° range of manipulation through a rotating handle with 4 uterine tip sizes, but can sometimes be difficult to place. The VCare uterine manipulator is a disposable, single-use device with a long, curved handle and a tip that conforms to the angle of the sacral curve. However, the fixed curve does not anteflex or retroflex across a joint. Both these devices offer several size colpotomy cups, which assist with lateral displacement of the ureters, anterior displacement of the bladder, and delineation of the cervicovaginal junction. The Pelosi uterine manipulator is a reusable device with 0° to 90° movement, which allows maximal anteversion of the uterus, and also has a long handle to maximize uterine elevation, although there is only 1 size colpotomy cup.

LESS Ports

Olympus America

The TriPort Access System from Olympus America (Center Valley, PA, USA) permits the placement of up to 3 laparoscopic instruments through a single incision of between 12 and 25 mm (**Fig. 1**). The QuadPort allows for up to 4 instruments. The system includes a plastic introducer that facilities the intra-abdominal placement of a flexible, inner ring. Once the introducer is through the incision, a switch is deployed

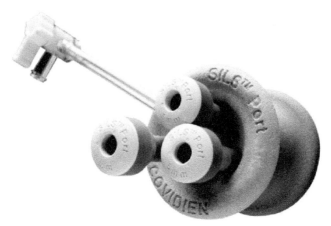

Fig. 2. SILS port (*Courtesy of* Covidien, Mansfield MA. © 2010 Covidien, All rights reserved. Used with permission of Covidien.).

that deposits the inner ring into the abdominal cavity. A second piece is then clamped across the upper ring. The instrument shafts can accommodate two 5-mm and one 12-mm instruments. It is recommended that the shafts be lubricated to ease the movement of the instruments. A removal ring is attached by a ribbon to the distal ring to facilitate removal of the port at the completion of the case.

Covidien, Inc.
The SILS port from Covidien (Norwalk, CT, USA) is a single-piece, flexible, marsh-mallow-shaped device made from a sponge-like elastic polymer (**Fig. 2**). It can accommodate three 5-mm instruments, or two 5-mm and one 5/12-mm port, and these ports can be interchanged throughout the case. The port is placed through a 20- to 25-mm incision. Once the incision has been made, a curved retractor (such as an "S" retractor) is placed within the inferior aspect of the incision and used to "shoe-horn" the port in place. The port can be removed and replaced throughout the case to facilitate specimen retrieval.

SurgiQuest
At first look, the AirSeal port from SurgiQuest (Orange, CT, USA) seems to be similar to any other rigid laparoscopic trocar (**Fig. 3**). Closer inspection, however, reveals the absence of an inner mechanical valve. Pneumoperitoneum is maintained by a pressure gradient created within the housing of the trocar. The pressure gradient exceeds the pressure created by the pneumoperitoneum. The system uses a specialized air pump and tubing, and the circulating air is filtered to help to remove smoke. Oddly shaped or traditional instruments may be passed through this device unencumbered.[16]

Karl Storz
The Karl Storz company (Tutlingen, Germany) refers to their LESS procedure instrumentation offerings as S-PORTAL products. These include a variety of long, specially curved instruments along with reusable peritoneal access ports. The X-Cone consists of 2 metal halves that, once within the peritoneal cavity, are joined together by a silicone cap (**Fig. 4**). Within the cap are 3 access channels that can accommo-date instruments up to 12-mm in diameter. It is inserted through a 2- to 2.5-cm

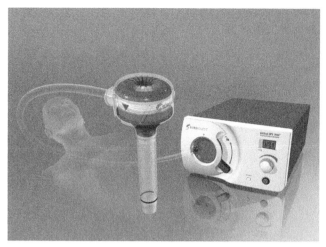

Fig. 3. Airseal port (*Courtesy of* SurgiQuest, Inc., Orange,CT; with permission.).

incision. The ENDOCONE requires a 3.5-cm incision,[17] but permits the passage of more instruments than any other currently available design. It contains channels for six 5-mm instruments and two 12-mm instruments.

Applied Medical

Utilizing the same materials present in their hand-assist port, Applied Medical (Rancho Santa Margarita, CA, USA) has created the GelPoint for use in LESS surgeries (**Fig. 5**). The GelPoint

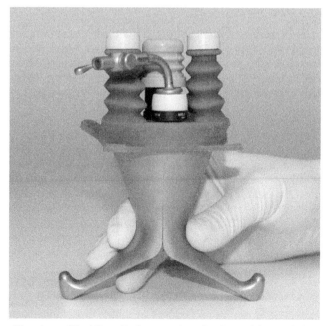

Fig. 4. X-cone (*Courtesy of* Karl Storz Endoscopy-America, Inc., with permission. © 2010 KARL STORZ Endoscopy-America, Inc.).

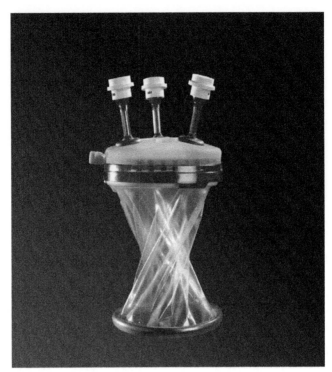

Fig. 5. GelPoint (*Courtesy of* Applied Medical Resources Corporation, Rancho Santa, CA; with permission.).

can be used in incisions ranging from 1.5 to 7 cm. It incorporates the company's Alexis wound retractor and the GelSeal cap. The GelSeal cap creates a PseudoAbdomen that floats above the fascial incision. This provides for a very flexible fulcrum around which the cannulae can move entirely independent of one another. This cap can be removed and replaced to facilitate specimen retrieval.

Ethicon endo-surgery

Also utilizing technology available in their hand-assist device, Ethicon Endo-Surgery (Cincinnati, OH, USA) has developed the Single Site Laparoscopy Access System (**Fig. 6**). This product consists of a seal cap that is fixed to an abdominal wall retractor. Because these wound retractors are fixed in size, there are 2 widths available from which to choose. The 2-cm width can be used in patients with and abdominal width of less than 4-cm. The 4-cm width can be used in patients with abdominal wall thicknesses between 4 and 7 cm. There are two 5-mm and one 5/15-mm channel present within the cap. The Single Site Laparoscopy system is placed through a 1.5- to 3.5-cm incision. An insertion tool is provided to facilitate placement of the fixed-length retractors.

Articulating Instrumentation

The challenges of LESS operative procedures, including loss of triangulation, reduced operative working space, and instrument collisions, can be partially mitigated with the use of articulating instrumentation. These instruments allow creation of an internal

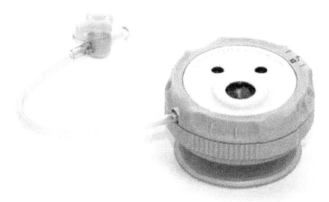

Fig. 6. Ethicon Single Site Laparoscopy port (*Courtesy of* Ethicon Endo-Surgery, Inc., Cincinatti, OH; with permission.).

type of triangulation, despite parallel instrument placement, that can assist the surgeon with appropriate tissue manipulation. Because instruments are typically introduced through a single, multichannel port during a LESS hysterectomy procedure, it is recommended that at least 1 or 2 articulating instruments be used during these procedures. Combined use of a flexible-tip laparoscope with articulating instruments seems to provide maximal flexibility. There are currently several articulating instruments available commercially for use in LESS hysterectomy procedures.

The Covidien Roticulator and SILS Hand Instruments (Covidien) are 5-mm laparoscopic instruments that provide articulating distal tips. The Covidien Roticulator provides up to an 80° articulating distal tip, with 360° rotation at all articulation angles. This instrument is not a fully articulating instrument because it does not articulate in all directions around the axis of the tip. The Roticulator comes in a dissector, shear, and grasper instruments. The SILS Hand instruments provide true articulation with the ability to lock the instrument in any position. These articulating instruments come in graspers, dissectors, shears, and a hook. Both instruments can be crossed intraperitoneally, and appropriately fixed at a specific articulation angle, to provide adequate triangulation during a LESS hysterectomy procedure. This can result in an opposing instrument handle and tip positions, meaning that the surgeon controls tissue on the opposite side from the external location of the instrument handle. This may require the surgeon to maximize use of their nondominant hand because their right hand may be controlling an instrument that is manipulating tissue on the left side and vice versa. Although this configuration is counterintuitive for a traditionally trained laparoscopic surgeon, this type of instrument and tissue manipulation is often necessary for effective performance of a LESS hysterectomy procedure.

Cambridge Endoscopic Devices (Framingham, MA, USA) are a line of 5-mm articulating instruments offering a Metzenbaum Scissors, Maryland dissector, electrocautery hook, fenestrated alligator grasper, and needle holder. These instruments are designed with a unique angled handle, an articulating distal tip with 360° axial rotation and 7 degrees of freedom with the ability to lock and rotate at any angle. The Spider Surgical System by TransEnterix is a unique newer device that enables true intra-abdominal triangulation achieved through a single-site port system. This system uses an expansion technology with true left and right instrumentation through flexible, articulating instruments with 360° range of motion. The Spider MicroLap instruments are

2.7-mm, reusable laparoscopic surgical instruments constructed of a ceramic titanium alloy shaft to maximize strength in a small diameter instrument.

Stryker (Kalamazoo, MI, USA) developed the ultrathin, 2.3-mm percutaneous MiniLap instruments, which enables the gynecologic surgeon to perform essentially "scar-less" surgical procedures while using the traditional techniques of multiport laparoscopy. The access insertion needle tip allows for percutaneous access without the need for a laparoscopic port, and the stainless steel instrumentation tip and stabilizing pivot disk provide strength with the ability to retract and manipulate tissue. These instruments come in a variety of clamps including Alligator, Babcock, clutch, and bowel clamps. This instrument allows the surgeon to preserve instrument triangulation while significantly limiting skin incision size, scarring, and pain.

Less Laparoscopes

Flexible-tip laparoscopes provide the surgeon with increased visualization during LESS hysterectomy procedures. The Olympus EndoEYE (Olympus Medical Systems, Tokyo, Japan) is a 5-mm flexible endoscope, with a distally mounted CCD chip and integrated light cable and camera system, that provides a 100° field of view deflectable distal tip. The Stryker IDEAL EYES HD is a 10-mm articulating endoscope that transmits both HD (1280 × 1024) and HDTV (720-p) video signals for enhanced visualization. The handle allows the surgeon to toggle between rigid and flexible-tip camera images, offers a friction-assist brake to fix the distal tip in position without the need for a locking mechanism, and provides over a 100° of flexion in all directions.

Flexible-tip laparoscopes are especially useful during a LESS hysterectomy procedure because they allow effective manipulation of the laparoscope to minimize instrument collisions. Because the surgical instruments are manipulated within the crowded space above and below the single incision port, there is a significant potential for instrument sword fighting (collisions) throughout the procedure. The flexible-tip laparoscope provides flexion at the distal tip, which allows the handle and rod of the laparoscope to be positioned against the patient's external abdominal wall, while the flexible tip is positioned up against the interior anterior abdominal wall and angled downward toward the operative site. This allows appropriate visualization during the procedure while remaining outside the crowded port space and out of the way of the laparoscopic instruments. Flexible-tip laparoscopes, therefore, provide significant flexibility and benefit over traditional rigid scopes. If flexible-tip laparoscopes are not available, then a 30° or 45° angled rigid bariatric scope with a right-angle light connector is preferred. These laparoscopes are not as versatile as flexible scopes, but do provide the surgeon with the ability to keep the camera out of the single-incision port working space.

Laparoscopic holders allow the surgeon to fix the laparoscope in a set position, while freeing up an extra hand, which may enable the surgeon the ability to operate more efficiently. This is especially important during LESS hysterectomy procedures, because the surgeon is required to manipulate multiple instruments within a confined space, while possibly controlling a uterine manipulator. The Stryker Wingman is a pneumatic-driven scope holding system that can be used to stabilize any 5- or 10-mm laparoscope and camera. The Wingman is especially useful to stabilize the flexible-tip laparoscopic handle against the exterior anterior abdominal wall, so that the laparoscope does not interfere with the surgical instruments positioned in the working space above and below the single-incision port, which improves efficient manipulation of these instruments. The flexible laparoscope can thus be fixed in a standard position during LESS hysterectomy procedures, because the tip deflection controls are located on the laparoscopic handle, which allows deflection of the tip in multiple directions and adjustment of visualization without moving the body of the laparoscope. The ViKY robotic laparoscope holder (Endocontrol Medical, La Tronche, France) is a robotic laparoscopic manipulator controlled through voice recognition or footswitch control. The FreeHand laparoscopic camera controller (Prosurgics, Cupertino, CA, USA) also gives the surgeons hands-free movement of the laparoscope using a robotic platform that uses surgeon head movement and an activation controller for manipulation.

SURGICAL TECHNIQUES IN LESS SURGERY

Gynecologic surgeons should not attempt to advance to LESS surgery until they are comfortable with multiport laparoscopy. There is a natural progression to minimize the number of port sites to a single port: First, after one has learned abdominal entry and trocar placement; second, after one has learned to view and understand the anatomy through a videolaparoscope; and third, after one has learned to triangulate and operate with instruments through multiple ports. Each of these steps needs to be modified or adapted when performing LESS surgery, but the confidence and skills of multiport laparoscopy provide a necessary foundation. In fact, if a situation arises where a LESS approach is limiting or inadequate, then an additional port (or several ports) can be added as necessary to complete the procedure. Multiport laparoscopy, then, is both the starting point and a backup plan for LESS surgery.

An open Hasson technique is used for abdominal entry at the umbilicus. The skin incision is strictly independent of the fascial incision or entry point. The umbilicus can vary greatly in women in size, depth, and shape. The skin incision, therefore, can be made to mimic the natural creases of the umbilicus in either a curved infraumbilical incision, also known as an "Omega"-type incision, as a linear incision, or as a "J"-shaped or "hockey-stick" incision. Most important, the goal is to make the incision such that there is no skin incision outside the edge of the umbilical crater. To avoid disfigurement of the umbilicus, it is best if the natural attachment of umbilical stalk is maintained, and if the fascia can be entered at the base of the where the stalk is attached. Once the fascia is entered, and this can be done so bluntly with a curved hemostat, the fascial defect can be extended in either the horizontal or vertical direction. Any of the available single-port systems can then be introduced per the manufacturer's recommendations.

Ideally, a flexible laparoscope is used during LESS surgery, which allows the camera head to stay near the abdominal wall and out of the way of the other instruments. A 5-mm, flexible laparoscope is preferable to a 10-mm laparoscope, which is more bulky. If a 5-mm, flexible laparoscope is unavailable, then an angled 45° laparoscope may be used; in this case, a bariatric length laparoscope is recommended with a 90° adaptor for the light post to deflect the light cord out of the way. Regardless of the laparoscope used, it is advantageous to be able to change the surgical view in LESS surgery by using the levers on the camera head for a flexible scope, or by moving the light post with an angled scope, as opposed to moving the entire camera head as with multiport laparoscopy. Minimizing camera head movement in LESS surgery is an important way to avoid instrument collisions.

Collisions of the instrument handles are the main frustration and obstacle for gynecologic surgeons who are comfortable with multiport laparoscopy as they move toward adopting LESS surgery. The main strategy for preventing collisions is to recreate triangulation by keeping all but the primary operating instrument away from the "target" zone. This "target" zone is the area midline in the axial direction, and in the highest height or plane above the abdominal wall.

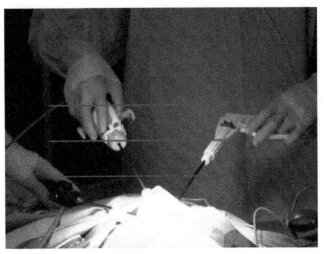

Fig. 7. Planes above the level of the patient. Note that each instrument resides in its own plane, the head of the laparoscope being in the most inferior plane and the energy source (surgeon's right hand) residing in the most superior plane.

Keeping the instrument handles away from each other is done deliberately and in a step-wise fashion during LESS surgery. The space above the abdominal wall can be thought of in different heights or planes (**Fig. 7**). Grasping instruments have been designed for LESS surgery that bend or articulate. These articulating instruments allow triangulation to be created at the surgical site intracorporeally, while maintaining the instrument handles apart extracorporeally. If the handles of the graspers—or instruments used for tissue retraction—are always retracted away from the midline (**Fig. 8**), in the middle height or plane above the abdominal wall, the main operating instrument (eg, the energy device) will be allowed to move in the "target" zone without collision. Unlike multiport laparoscopy, it is also helpful to minimize simultaneous movements of the instruments in LESS surgery, and to move only 1 instrument at a time to avoid collisions.

Once triangulation in LESS surgery has been created, and the instruments handles made to be apart, the steps for any procedure are essentially the same as for multiport hysterectomy.

LEARNING CURVE

An important aspect in the adoption of LESS surgery is to have a reasonable expectation of the learning curve. It is recommended that training first occur on dry, then animal, labs to be comfortable with the port placement, instrumentation, and techniques involved in LESS surgery before proceeding to human cases.[17,18] Recent studies[18,19] have shown that it takes between 10 and 20 cases to significantly decrease operative times and achieve proficiency. (Of note, in the general surgery literature, the learning curve for LESS cholecystectomy was overcome in as few as 8 cases.[20]) It is expected that this learning phase is needed to learn to place the ports in the umbilicus with ease, to become comfortable with the new instrumentation, and to learn the LESS surgical techniques needed for adequate tissue retraction and triangulation. It is important to note that these studies did not show an increase in complications during the time that proficiency was achieved. (Another study in the

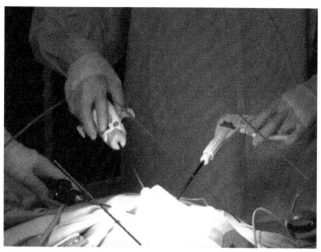

Fig. 8. Planes from midline to lateral. Note that each instrument resides in its own plane, the head of the laparoscope being in the most medial plane and the articulating grasper (surgeon's left hand) residing in the most lateral plane.

general surgery literature, which evaluated the learning curve for LESS cholecystectomy, showed that there was no increased rate of complications nor an increase in conversion rates in successive cohorts of 25 patients, at least in surgeons skilled at multiport laparoscopy.[21] Thus, the learning phase of LESS surgery is shorter, and with less morbidity, than the expectation for learning other multiport laparoscopic procedures (about 25 cases).[22,23] Thus, the adoption of LESS surgery by surgeons familiar with multiport laparoscopy may be achieved in a relatively efficient manner, without increased risk to the patient.

EVIDENCE FOR BENEFIT OF LESS PROCEDURES IN GYNECOLOGY

When considering the potential advantages of operating through a single umbilical incision, there are several benefits that could be imagined. The first, and perhaps most obvious advantage, is cosmetic. As described, it is possible to limit the incision to entirely within the confines of the umbilical crater thus making it virtually invisible (**Fig. 9**). Bush and colleagues[24] have shown that when compared with the typical location of robotic surgery port site incisions, patients preferred the location of incisions typically utilized in both conventional and LESS laparoscopic procedures.

In addition to a cosmetic advantage, limiting the number and location of the incisions to the umbilicus may result in less postoperative pain. There are 3 published comparative trials studying the differences between multiport and single-port laparoscopic hysterectomy. In 2010, Kim and colleagues[25] published a retrospective review comparing LESS–LAVH cases performed between May 2008 and February 2009 with a series of control multiport LAVH patients from 2005 to 2008. There were 43 patients in each arm of the study. To provide instrument access for the patients in the single-incision group, the surgeons in the study devised a novel "port" system that involved placing a small Alexis wound retractor (Applied Medical) through the umbilical incision. The wrist portion of a surgical glove was then wrapped around the wound retractor so that pneumoperitoneum could be maintained. After making a small hole into the tip of one of the fingers of the glove, standard 5-mm or 10- to

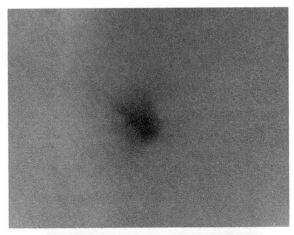

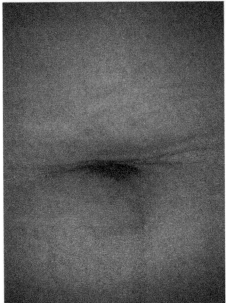

Fig. 9. Umbilical incisions at 6 weeks.

11-mm trocars were placed through the holes in the fingertips and these and could be used for instrument placement. The operative time, blood loss, and drop in hemoglobin were comparable between groups. VAS pain scores measured at 24 hours (2.5 vs 3.5; $P<.01$) and at 36 hours (1.7 vs 2.9; $P<.01$) after surgery were significantly lower in the LESS–LAVH group. Scores taken at 12 hours after surgery were similar between groups.

Also in 2010, Yim and colleagues[26] published their retrospective review of 52 women who underwent a LESS TLH with 105 women who underwent traditional TLH. This group utilized a similar umbilical access system as in the study described. There was less blood loss, larger uterine weight, and a shorter hospital stay for the LESS hysterectomy patients. There was no difference in mean operative time or perioperative complications between groups. Pain scores were measured immediately postoperatively in the recovery room, and at 6, 24, and 48 hours after surgery. Patients who underwent LESS-TLH had significantly lower pain scores in the immediate postoperative time period than those who underwent multiport procedures (3.5 vs 4.5; $P<$ .001). Although scores were lower for LESS-TLH patients at 6 and 24 hours, they did not attain significance. Pain scores at 48 hours were the same between groups.

Finally, Chen and colleagues[27] published a randomized, controlled trial comparing LESS-LAVH with conventional LAVH procedures. In this study, 50 patients were randomly assigned to each group. Based on their initial pilot study,[25] this trial was adequately powered to demonstrate a pain difference between the groups. This was a single-surgeon, single-institution study. Once again, there were no differences between the groups when operative times, blood loss, or length of stay were compared. The LESS-LAVH group had significantly lower pain scores at 24 hours (VAS 3.64 vs 5.08; $P = $ .011) and at 48 hours (VAS 1.94 vs 2.84; $P = $ .043). This resulted in the use of significantly lower total amounts of postoperative analgesics (74.40 vs 104.80 mg meperidine; $P = $ .001).

FUTURE DIRECTION FOR LESS GYNECOLOGY PROCEDURES

The field of LESS surgery is currently in its infancy, but is rapidly maturing as newer technologies and instrumentation have become available. Although the first case of a single-incision laparoscopic hysterectomy was reported approximately 20 years ago,[10] adoption of this type of procedure has not been possible until the last several years because of the rapid introduction of newer technologies and instrumentation within the field of minimally invasive surgery. The success of LESS surgery will increasingly depend on technology, and the ability of industry to develop newer and more innovative devices specifically designed to enable surgeons to perform these complex procedures.

Articulating laparoscopes and instruments will continue to play an increasingly important role in LESS gynecologic surgery. Intra-abdominal instrument articulation is essential to recreate the basic principles of triangulation, which is lost during LESS surgery, and is essential for effective and efficient performance of laparoscopic procedures. Articulating laparoscopes allow flexible visualization within the confined space beneath the single incision laparoscopic port in the abdomen. Introduction of articulating energy devices will permit tissue cautery, sealing, and transection without the need for significant tissue manipulation. Articulating instruments can also reduce port site trauma, which can be caused by excessive torquing of straight instruments owing to the midline entry, and required manipulation of these instruments to accommodate for unfavorable tissue angles. Innovative delivery systems in the future may also allow single or multiple instruments to be inserted through a single laparoscopic incision, and then separated to create adequate triangulation, but allow manipulation in a natural and intuitive manner.

Alternatively, development of smaller diameter laparoscopic instruments may allow traditional multiport laparoscopic surgery to be performed without the scarring or discomfort currently encountered from traditional 5- to 12-mm laparoscopic ports. These instruments have the potential to preserve the technique of triangulation, while reducing the size of the skin incision and subsequent scar formation. Instruments, such as the Stryker MiniLap graspers or TransEnterix Spider MicroLap instruments, may eventually allow surgeons to perform a traditional multiport TLH with minimal to no visible scars.

Advanced technologies will undoubtedly have a role in reducing many of the challenges currently encountered during LESS surgical procedures. Robotic surgical platforms can potentially eliminate the difficulties associated with instrument crowding and collision caused by reduced operative working space, as well as enable compensation for the opposite-sided tissue control currently necessary to perform efficient LESS operative procedures. Innovative medical technologies such as magnetic anchoring systems to control intra-abdominal cameras and operative instruments from outside the abdominal wall could also mitigate some of these challenges associated with LESS surgical procedures.[28]

These current laparoscopic devices, and newer innovative technologies, will help to reduce the steep learning curve, and high level of dexterity, currently necessary to perform these procedures. As LESS surgical procedures continue to develop, it will also become increasingly important to develop training programs for residents, fellows, and practicing physicians so that these techniques are adequately taught. The future of LESS surgery will continue to depend on technology, and industry partners, to provide surgeons with the innovative surgical equipment necessary to reduce the challenges associated with LESS procedures, and allow these surgical procedures to become more attainable for the majority of surgeons.

REFERENCES

1. Johnson N, Barlow D, Lethaby A, et al. Surgical approach to hysterectomy for benign gynaecological disease [review]. Cochrane Database Syst Rev 2006;192:CD003677.
2. Garry R, Fountain J, Brown J, et al. EVALUATE hysterectomy trial: a multicentre randomised trial comparing abdominal, vaginal, and laparoscopic methods of hysterectomy. Health Technol Assess 2004;8(26):1–154.
3. Kluivers KB, Hendricks JC, Mol BW, et al. Quality of life and surgical outcome after total laparoscopic hysterectomy versus total abdominal hysterectomy for benign disease: a randomized controlled trial. J Minim Invasiv Gynecol 2007;14:145–52.
4. Hulka JF, Levy BS, Parker WH, et al. Laparoscopic-assisted vaginal hysterectomy: American Association of Gynecologic Laparoscopicsts' 1995 member survey. J Am Assoc Gynecol Laparosc 1997;4:167–71.
5. Huang M, Musa F, Castillo C, et al. Postoperative bowel herniation in a 5-mm nonbladed trocar site. JSLS 2010;14:289–91.
6. Romanelli JR, Earle DB. Single-port laparoscopic surgery: an overview. Surg Endosc 2009;23:1419–27.
7. Gill IS, Advincula AP, Aron M, et al. Consensus statement of the consortium for laparoendoscopic single-site surgery. Surg Endosc 2010;24:762–8.
8. Wheeless CR, A rapid, inexpensive and effective method of surgical sterilization by laparoscopy. J Reprod Med 1969;3:65–9.
9. Wheeless CR, Jr, Thompson BH. Laparoscopic sterilization. Review of 3600 cases. Obstet Gynecol 1973;42:751–8.
10. Pelosi MA, Pelosi MA III. Laparoscopic hysterectomy with bilateral salpingo-oophorectomy using a single umbilical puncture. N Engl J Med 1991;88:721–6.
11. Pelosi MA. Single puncture laparoscopic sling procedure. J Am Assoc Gynecol Laparosc 1994;1:S28.
12. Pelosi MA, Pelosi MA 3rd. Laparoscopic supracervical hysterectomy using a single-umbilical puncture (mini-laparoscopy). J Reprod Med 1992;37:777–84.
13. Pelosi MA, Pelosi MA III. Laparoscopic appendectomy using a single umbilical puncture (minilaparoscopy). J Reprod Med 1992;37:588–94.
14. Wolenski M, Pelosi MA. The single puncture approach for advanced pelviscopy surgery. Todays OR Nurse 1991;13:4–8.
15. Rawlings A, Hodgett S, Matthews B, et al. Single-incision laparoscopic cholecystectomy: initial experience with critical review of safety dissection and routine intraoperative cholangiography. J Am Coll Surg 2010;211:1–7.

16. Raman J, Cadeddu J, Rao P, et al. Single-incision laparoscopic surgery: initial urological experience and comparison with natural-orifice transluminal endoscopic surgery. BJU Int 2008;101:1493–6.
17. Muller EM, Cavazzola LT, Machado Grossi JV, et al. Training for laparoendoscopic single-site surgery (LESS). Int J Surg 2010;8:64–8.
18. Escobar PF, Starks DC, Fader AN, et al. Single-port risk-reducing salpingo-oophorectomy with and without hysterectomy: surgical outcomes and learning curve analysis. Gynecol Oncol 2010;119:43–7.
19. Fader AN, Rojas-Espaillat L, Ibeanu O, et al. Laparoendoscopic single-site surgery (LESS) in gynecology: a multi-institutional evaluation. Am J Obstet Gynecol 2010;203: 501.
20. Han HJ, Choi SB, Park MS, et al. Learning curve of single port laparoscopic cholecystectomy determined using the non-linear ordinary least squares method based on a non-linear regression model: an analysis of 150 consecutive patients. J Hepatobiliary Pancreat Sci 2011;18:510–5.
21. Hernandez J, Ross S, Morton C, et al. The learning curve of laparoendoscopic single-site (LESS) cholecystectomy: definable, short, and safe. J Am Coll Surg 2010;211:652–7.
22. Schlachta CM, Mamazza J, Seshadri PA, et al. Defining a learning curve for laparoscopic colorectal resections. Dis Colon Rectum 2001;44:217–22.
23. Reade C, Hauspy J, Schmuck ML, et al. Characterizing the learning curve for laparoscopic radical hysterectomy: buddy operating as a technique for accelerating skill acquisition. Int J Gynecol Cancer 2011;21:930–5.
24. Bush AJ, Morris SN, Isaacson KB. Women's preferences for different minimally invasive incisions. J Minim Invas Gynecol 2011;17:S1–S2.
25. Kim TJ, Lee YY, Cha HH, et al. Single-port-access laparoscopic-assisted vaginal hysterectomy versus conventional laparoscopic-assisted vaginal hysterectomy: a comparison of perioperative outcomes. Surg Endosc 2010;24:2248–52.
26. Yim GA, Jung WJ, Paek J, et al. Transumbilical single-port access versus conventional total laparoscopic hysterectomy: surgical outcomes. Am J Obstet Gynecol 2010;203:e1–6.
27. Chen YJ, Wnag, PH, Ocampo EJ, et al. Single-port compared with conventional laparoscopic-assisted vaginal hysterectomy: a randomized controlled trial. Obstet Gynecol 2011;117:906–12.
28. Best SL, Cadeddu JA. Use of magnetic anchoring and guidance systems to facilitate single trocars laparoscopy. Curr Urol Rep 2010;11:29–32.

Laparoscopy in Pregnancy and the Pediatric Patient

Shan Biscette, MD, Jennie Yoost, MD, Paige Hertweck, MD, Jonathan Reinstine, MD*

KEYWORDS

- Laparoscopic surgery • Pediatrics • Pregnancy
- Adolescents • Endometriosis • Adnexal masses • Ovarian torsion • Mullerian anomalies

Laparoscopy is considered standard of care in the treatment of certain pathology in the pediatric and adolescent populations, such as endometriosis resection, ovarian cystectomy, and ovarian detorsion. Specific mullerian anomalies can also be managed laparoscopically. There are emerging data that laparoscopic oophoropexy gives favorable results in patients being treated for childhood malignancies to preserve ovarian function, and can expedite oncologic treatment compared with laparotomy. Single-incision laparoscopy is being investigated in children, but may prove beneficial for certain procedures. This article discusses the laparoscopic approach to treatment of abdominal diseases during pregnancy and in the pediatric patient.

Laparoscopy was considered to be absolutely contraindicated in pregnancy until 1990. Nezhat and colleagues[1] reported the first laparoscopic cystectomy in pregnancy in 1991. Since then, there has been an increase in these procedures as the safety of the technique in the pregnant population has been more widely appreciated.

LAPAROSCOPY IN PREGNANCY
Indications for Surgery in Pregnancy

Appendectomy

The most common nonobstetric emergency in pregnancy is acute appendicitis. The incidence during pregnancy is equal to that seen in the nonpregnant female population and is approximately 1 in 1500.[2] The largest hospital-based series of pregnant patients undergoing surgery for clinical suspicion of appendicitis was published by Sadot and associates in 2009.[3] The aim was to evaluate laparoscopic versus open surgery for suspected appendicitis. Sixty-five patients underwent surgery, 48 were treated laparoscopically, and 17 with an open approach. No difference was

Conflicts of Interest: Paige Hertweck, MD, receives research support and serves on the Speakers Bureau for Merck.

Department of Obstetrics, Gynecology and Women's Health, Kosair Children's Hospital, 4121 Dutchman's Lane, Suite 300, Louisville, KY 40207, USA

* Corresponding author.

E-mail address: Jreinstine@aol.com

Obstet Gynecol Clin N Am 38 (2011) 757–776
doi:10.1016/j.ogc.2011.10.001
0889-8545/11/$ – see front matter © 2011 Published by Elsevier Inc.

obgyn.theclinics.com

Table 1
Mean gestational age at the time of intervention and hospital length of stay

	Laparoscopic	Open
Mean gestational age (wk)	18.1	24.3
Length of hospital stay (d)	3.4	4.2
Surgical approach by trimester		
First	14	0
Second	32	12
Third	2	5

observed in the rate of advanced appendicitis between the laparoscopic and open approaches. Significance was noted between the laparoscopic and open groups with regard to mean gestational age at the time of intervention and hospital length of stay (**Table 1**). No significance was demonstrated between the 2 groups with regard to operative time, anesthesia time, mode of delivery, postoperative complications, and fetal outcomes. The overall preterm delivery rate and the 1-month preterm birth rate (defined as delivery within 1 month of the surgery) were equivalent. One fetal loss occurred in the laparoscopy group 10 weeks after the procedure and was thought to be a result of chorioamnionitis. The overall negative appendectomy rate was 24% with no difference noted between the 2 operative approaches. Although no significance was noted, the rate in the laparoscopy group was higher than the open approach (27% vs 18%). The authors concluded that this difference may reflect a trend toward early investigation with laparoscopy, as being considered safer than observation and reevaluation. This management approach may increase the negative appendectomy rate, but decrease the perforation rate.

Cholecystectomy
The second most common nonobstetric surgery performed during pregnancy is cholecystectomy for symptomatic cholelithiasis or advanced biliary disease.[4] Approximately 1 in 1600 pregnancies are complicated by these conditions. Patel and co-workers[5] performed a retrospective study of 10 patients undergoing cholecystectomy during pregnancy to evaluate the safety of the laparoscopic approach.[5] Eight out of 10 patients underwent the laparoscopic procedure and the other 2 had an open approach. Laparoscopy was performed in 6 patients in the second trimester and 2 in the first. No complications occurred in the 2 women treated in the first trimester and both delivered at term. Of the 2 patients who underwent laparotomy for treatment, 1 patient had a pregnancy loss in the first trimester and the other was lost to follow-up.

Review of the evidence-based literature has shown that when compared with open cholecystectomy, the laparoscopic approach has equivalent outcomes with decreased risk of spontaneous abortions and preterm labor.[6]

Adnexal masses
The diagnosis of abnormal adnexal masses is made in approximately 1 in 81 to 1 in 2200 pregnancies with an average of 1 in 600.[7] The frequency of ovarian cysts in pregnancy is 1 in 1000 pregnancies. The most frequently encountered ovarian tumors during pregnancy are mature cystic teratomas, which account for up to 50% of ovarian masses.[8,9] Functional cysts (13%), benign cystadenomas (20%), and ovarian cancer (0.6%) are the most frequent histologic types reported.[10]

Several authors have demonstrated successful laparoscopic removal of very large ovarian masses.[10,11] Some authors advocate observation of ovarian cystic masses greater than 6 cm if they seem to be benign and are asymptomatic.[9] The risks of observation versus the risks of surgery must be considered when counseling the patient. Patients with adnexal masses managed conservatively are at risk for ovarian torsion, cyst rupture with the potential for hemorrhage, infection, peritonitis, and obstruction of labor. The risk of undiagnosed malignancy is also cause for concern.[12]

Adnexal torsion has an incidence of 1 in 5000 in pregnancy. Its presentation in the first trimester is usually a result of ovarian stimulation for treatment of infertility. The clinical presentation is often nonspecific and may mimic other acute abdominal conditions. Doppler ultrasonography may aid in preoperative diagnosis; however, the gravid uterus may obscure the adnexa and limit its use. Laparotomy was traditionally used to evaluate and treat this condition; however, laparoscopy has proven useful both in diagnosis and treatment with adnexal detorsion or cystectomy.[13,14]

Laparoscopic removal of adnexal masses in pregnancy is safe and feasible.[9,12] Stepp and colleagues[12] performed a retrospective study to assess the safety of laparoscopic treatment of adnexal masses in the second trimester of pregnancy. Eleven women at 13 to 23 weeks of pregnancy had nonemergent laparoscopic management of adnexal masses ranging from 4 to 20 cm. Various trocar entry methods were used with left upper quadrant direct entry performed in 7 cases. Cysts were aspirated in 4 patients with masses larger than 14 cm before removal of the specimen. Pathology results showed no findings of malignancy in the study group. No intraoperative or postoperative complications were encountered. Several patients underwent various tocolytic agents for management of contractions; however, no patients had evidence of preterm labor and all were delivered at term.[12]

Yuen and co-workers[15] reported on one of the largest retrospective case series performed at a single institution evaluating the safety of laparoscopic management for persistent adnexal mass in the second trimester. Sixty-seven patients had laparoscopic removal of adnexal masses that persisted beyond the first trimester. Fifty-five women had ovarian cystectomies, 9 had oophorectomies, and 3 had fenestration. Two women had conversion to laparotomy, one for adhesions associated with a large endometrioma, and the other for a dermoid cyst adherent to the pouch of Douglas. All patients received general anesthesia. Abdominal entry was via an open entry technique through a supraumbilical incision and pneumoperitoneum was maintained at 12 mmHg using carbon dioxide. There were no intraoperative complications. No women experienced uterine contractions or received tocolysis. One patient had a pregnancy loss at 22 weeks, which occurred 6 weeks after the initial procedure to remove a dermoid cyst. Four patients had preterm delivery at 33 to 36 weeks' gestation. No fetal anomalies were observed. The authors of this study recommend that the open laparoscopy method be the standard for primary trocar entry to eliminate the potential risk of injury of the uterus associated with blind entry techniques. Supraumbilical primary port placement 6 cm above the uterine fundus is recommended to allow adequate visualization of the target organs and for ease of manipulation of instruments.

Advantages

Several authors have shown that the advantages of laparoscopy in the nonpregnant patient can be applied to the pregnant patient.[7] The laparoscope provides a magnified, improved, and wide view of the operative field. The smaller incisions used to gain access into the abdomen result in lesser postoperative pain and a more rapid postoperative recovery. Reduced postoperative pain leads to a decreased need for postoperative narcotics, earlier ambulation, and a reduction in risk of thromboembolism. Fetal depression is also less likely with reduced maternal narcotic use. Bowel manipulation is minimal during laparoscopy, which aids in a quicker return to bowel function, and a possible decrease in postoperative adhesions, ileus, and bowel obstruction.[16-18] The smaller scars seen with laparoscopy result in fewer incisional hernias, lower risk of wound complications, and less opportunity for wound dehiscence as the uterus grows and distends the abdomen. Patients undergoing laparoscopic procedures also have a shorter hospital stay and a prompt return to regular activities.[19]

Physiology and anesthesia

Pneumoperitoneum is essential for visualization and performance of laparoscopic procedures. The cardiovascular and respiratory alterations observed with pneumoperitoneum during laparoscopy are accentuated in the pregnant patient as compared with the general population.[20] The mechanical displacement of the diaphragm by the enlarging uterus coupled with pneumoperitoneum is associated with decreased compliance of the thoracic cavity, a decrease in the functional reserve capacity, an increase in peak airway pressure, ventilation–perfusion mismatching, increased alveolar–arterial oxygen gradient, and increased pleural pressure. These changes are further accentuated by the Trendelenburg position commonly employed in laparoscopy.[20-22] The partial pressure of arterial carbon dioxide is increased with pneumoperitoneum as a result of absorption of carbon dioxide from the peritoneal cavity. There is concern that this increase and the concomitant decrease in arterial pH may adversely affect the fetus because fetal arterial CO_2 is directly related to maternal arterial CO_2. Bhavani-Shankar and associates[23] investigated this issue in 8 pregnant women at 17 to 24 weeks' gestation undergoing laparoscopic surgery with carbon dioxide pneumoperitoneum. The minute ventilation was adjusted to keep the end tidal CO_2 at 32 mmHg and arterial blood gas was measured at preinsufflation, insufflation, postinsufflation, and postoperatively. No differences were observed in the partial pressure of arterial CO_2 to end-tidal CO_2 gradient, or the partial pressure of arterial CO_2 and pH during the various phases of monitoring. The authors concluded that end-tidal CO_2 correlated with arterial CO_2 and that optimal maternal arterial CO_2 could be maintained during laparoscopy by adjusting minute ventilation. Blood gas monitoring may not be necessary in healthy patients undergoing laparoscopy.[23]

Cardiovascular and hemodynamic changes associated with pneumoperitoneum result from the combination of the physiologic effects of patient positioning, anesthesia, and carbon dioxide absorption. Insufflation causes a decrease in cardiac output, with a concurrent increase in systemic and pulmonary vascular resistance and blood pressure.[20,21] The reverse Trendelenburg position has been shown to exacerbate the cardiovascular changes seen with general anesthesia and pneumoperitoneum with a reduction in the cardiac index of up to 50%. Significant hypotension is also observed as a result of aortocaval compression by the pregnant uterus coupled with the other cardiovascular changes induced by pneumoperitoneum.[20,21] One study investigating the hemodynamic changes in laparoscopic surgery in pregnant women showed that cardiac index dropped to 21% below baseline after 15 minutes of insufflation. Systolic blood pressure 20% below baseline was aggressively managed with intravenous ephedrine in an effort to minimize any decrease in uterine perfusion.[23] Left uterine displacement and limiting the intra-abdominal insufflation pressure to 12 to 15 mmHg are essential to minimizing these cardiovascular changes.[23]

Operative Techniques

Controversies regarding laparoscopy during pregnancy include timing, the safest method of abdominal cannulation, and appropriate fetal and maternal monitoring. The first trimester of pregnancy poses the least technical difficulty during abdominal and pelvic surgery. The uterus is well below the point of initial trocar entry and visualization of the pelvis and adnexa is optimal. The potential for teratogenesis, however, is greatest during this trimester. Surgery performed in the second trimester of pregnancy poses less risk to the fetus; however, it is technically more difficult and requires greater surgical skill. The third trimester is associated with a greater potential for preterm labor and the issue of visualization noted in the second trimester is further pronounced by the enlarging uterus. Because the rate of spontaneous abortion decreases and the rate of premature labor increases as pregnancy progresses, it seems obvious that the second trimester is the safest interval for operative intervention for elective cases.[16]

The placement of the laparoscope and operating trocars is determined by uterine size and gestational age. The open Hasson technique is used by a majority of surgeons when performing surgery in the second and third trimesters; however, studies have indicated that a closed entry technique is undertaken by others.[24] When using the Veress needle for insufflation in the closed entry technique, a left upper quadrant (Palmer's point) entry is often used beyond the first trimester. In this method, the primary trocar is placed in the midclavicular line, 2 cm below the ribcage. Ultrasound guidance can further improve the safety of Veress needle and trocar insertion. Alternatively, a subxyphoid entry can be performed with the trocar placement 2 to 6 cm above the umbilicus, depending on the fundal height. Secondary trocars are then placed under direct visualization. Vaginal instrumentation, cervical clamps, and uterine manipulators should be avoided in the pregnant patient.[25]

Optimal perioperative monitoring is unclear given the large number of physiologic changes seen in pregnancy and the cardiovascular and pulmonary changes induced by laparoscopic surgery. The usual precautions applied to pregnant women undergoing surgery should be upheld in laparoscopic surgery. End-tidal CO_2 should be maintained between 32 and 34 mmHg when using CO_2 insufflation by increasing respiratory rate and tidal volume and systolic blood pressure should be kept within 20% of baseline.[21]

The concern for the effects of CO_2 pneumoperitoneum has prompted the use of an apneumatic approach by some surgeons. With this method, laparoscopy is performed under epidural anesthesia and abdominal access is achieved by mechanical lifting of the abdominal wall with wire spokes.[26,27] Although this method eliminates the effects of carbon dioxide insufflation seen with general endotracheal anesthesia and is an appealing option for patients with preexisting cardiopulmonary disease, further research is necessary to validate its efficacy.

With regard to fetal monitoring, studies have shown no intraoperative fetal heart rate abnormalities. In the setting of urgent abdominal surgery during pregnancy, fetal monitoring is considered to be sufficient in the pre- and postoperative periods. No increased fetal morbidity has been reported with this approach.[6]

Patient positioning is important in laparoscopic procedures. Visualization of pelvic organs can be difficult because of the obstruction by the bowel and omentum, the gravid uterus, and maternal obesity. Trendelenburg positioning is essential for laparoscopic pelvic surgeries, whereas the reverse Trendelenberg is utilized in upper abdominal surgeries. The patient should be placed in supine position with a leftward tilt to minimize further compression of the inferior vena cava by the uterus, thereby maximizing venous return to the heart and uterine perfusion. When using the Trendelenberg position, any changes should be gradual to reduce the effect on hemodynamic stability.

The Society of American Gastrointestinal Endoscopic Surgeons Guidelines for Laparoscopic Surgery during Pregnancy recommends the following.[28]

- Gravid patients should be placed in the left lateral decubitus position to minimize compression of the vena cava.
- Initial abdominal access can be safely performed with an open (Hasson) technique, Veress needle, or optical trocar if the location is adjusted according to fundal height and previous incisions.
- Intraoperative CO_2 monitoring by capnography should be used during laparoscopy in the pregnant patient.
- Intraoperative and postoperative pneumatic compression devices and early postoperative ambulation are recommended prophylaxis for deep venous thrombosis in the gravid patient.
- Fetal heart monitoring should occur pre- and postoperatively in the setting of urgent abdominal surgery during pregnancy.
- Obstetric consultation can be obtained pre- and/or postoperatively based on the severity of the patient's disease and availability.
- Tocolytics should not be used prophylactically in pregnant women undergoing surgery, but should be considered perioperatively when signs of preterm labor are present.

Outcomes

The lack of prospective trials and the understudied risks of laparoscopy in pregnancy have prevented the extrapolation of the success of laparoscopy in the general population to the pregnant population. Laparoscopic procedures have been safely performed on pregnant women for decades. Women suspected of having ectopic pregnancies with subsequent finding of normal first trimester pregnancies have progressed to normal gestation and birth.

Rizzo[29] evaluated the effects of laparoscopic procedures during pregnancy with patient and child follow-up during a 1- to 8-year period. Eleven pregnant women underwent laparoscopic procedures with only 1 conversion to laparotomy. The surgeries were performed in the first through third trimesters of pregnancy (10–28 weeks) for acute cholecystitis, chronic cholecystitis and biliary colic, appendicitis, and bowel obstruction. The operative protocol was similar for all patients. All patients had general anesthesia, an open Hasson entry technique, end-tidal CO_2 monitoring, insufflations pressure of 10 mmHg, and left lateral positioning. Operative time ranged from 25 to 90 minutes. Postoperative fetal monitoring was performed for a total of 24 hours. No fetal distress, need for tocolysis, or fetal demise was observed. The patients and their offspring were followed for 6 years. No medical issues or failure to thrive were observed in the offspring.[29]

A much earlier study by Amos and colleagues[30] had raised concerns about the effect of CO_2 pneumoperitoneum and laparoscopy in the fetus. The study compared the pregnancy outcomes for 7 women managed with laparoscopic surgery with 5 patients who had laparotomy (**Table 2**). In the laparoscopic group, the procedure was performed for urgent and emergent indications for diagnoses of gallstone pancreatitis, acute cholecystitis, and acute appendicitis with 1 instance of gross perforation. Four fetal losses occurred in the laparoscopic group (3 in the immediate postpartum period and another 4 weeks later); none occurred in the laparotomy group. Even

Table 2
Pregnancy outcomes for 7 women managed laparoscopically and 5 patients who underwent laparotomy

	n	Cholecystectomy	Appendectomy	Adnexal Surgery	Fetal Loss	Patients Lost to Follow-Up
Laparoscopy	7	4	3	0	Two intrauterine death; 2 incomplete abortions	0
Laparotomy	5	0	0	5	0	1

though the nature of the surgical pathologies were significantly different between the 2 groups, the authors contended that clinical stability had been observed in several patients before surgery, and maintained that laparoscopy and CO_2 pneumoperitoneum may have contributed to the outcomes observed. Other authors have challenged the validity of these claims and postulate that the fetal loss seen in this group was more likely a consequence of the severity of the illness rather than the operative procedure itself.[25,29]

Animal studies have been done to evaluate the effects of laparoscopy on maternal and fetal physiology, especially in regard to pneumoperitoneum.[31] The small experimental numbers of these studies limit interpretation of the results observed; however, they do reveal some trends. Sheep studies evaluating the effects of CO_2 and helium insufflation on maternal and fetal blood gas status showed that insufflation with CO_2 produced maternal and fetal acidosis and a prolonged rise in fetal blood lactate concentration. The fetal effects persisted beyond those of the mother, even after deflation of CO_2 gas. Fetal blood oxygen status was not affected by CO_2 insufflation.[31] This and other animal studies show collectively that CO_2 insufflation during laparoscopy is capable of producing maternal and fetal hypercarbia; however, as long as maternal oxygenation is maintained, no adverse fetal effects ensue. Studies of human subjects do not demonstrate the findings seen in animal studies.[23]

Pregnancy is sometimes complicated by diseases necessitating operative intervention. A growing body of evidence indicates that laparoscopic surgery can be safely performed with marked benefits for patients.

LAPAROSCOPY IN PEDIATRIC GYNECOLOGY
Approach to the Pediatric Patient

Special considerations must be made for pediatric and adolescent gynecology patients undergoing laparoscopy. In the operating room, positioning of the patient is critical. Allen stirrups can be used to position a pediatric patient if they are tall enough. Smaller patients can be placed in the frog-leg position with supportive gel pads. If vaginal preparation is needed, a sponge stick in prep solution can be used. If there is a tight introitus, or in virginal patients, the use of a Toomey syringe filled with prep solution introduced through the hymen has been described.[32]

Uterine manipulation can be accomplished by digital manipulation, or if the introitus is large enough, by use of a sponge stick. A tenaculum and cervical dilator affixed together have also been described.[32] In adolescent patients, commercial uterine manipulators are most helpful.

Abdominal entry can be achieved by use of a Veress needle, direct trocar entry, or direct visual entry using a Visiport or Optiview trocar in which the laparoscope is used with in the trocar to visualize the layers as the abdomen is entered. Open entry technique with placement of a Hassan trocar can also be used. A Cochrane review of the literature showed no advantages of 1 technique over another, but the studies reviewed were all performed on adult patients.[33] Pediatric patients are often thin and, regardless of entry method, it is important to recall the small distance between the umbilicus and the pelvic brim to avoid entry-related injuries to large vessels or the bowel.

The amount of intra-abdominal insufflation to obtain pneumoperitoneum is based on size of the patient, body habitus, and abdominal wall distensibility. Infants can tolerate 6 to 8 mmHg, children 8 to 10 mmHg, and older children and adolescents 10 to 15 mmHg. Patients with cardiac or pulmonary comorbidities can also affect the amount of pneumoperitoneum. Most children, however, can tolerate transient increases of up to 25 mmHg to facilitate port placement.[32]

Endometriosis

Laparoscopy can be an integral part of managing endometriosis in an adolescent patient. Endometriosis is defined by the presence of endometrial glands and stroma outside the uterus. This diagnosis can only be made via histopathology of a biopsy specimen. Adolescents with endometriosis present with cyclic and/or acyclic pain, and dysmenorrhea. The pain is usually disruptive and interferes with school, sports, and other social activities. Abnormal bleeding accompanied by cramping is related to increased prostaglandin formation by endometrial implants.[34]

The incidence of endometriosis in adolescents varies from 19% to 73% in those undergoing laparoscopy for chronic pelvic pain.[35] It has been shown that 70% of adolescent girls with pelvic pain not responsive to combination hormone therapy have endometriosis at the time of laparoscopy.[36] First-degree relatives of patients with endometriosis have a 6.9% incidence of endometriosis compared with a 1% risk in controls.[37]

Atypical endometriotic lesions include clear papules, red flame-like lesions, and white lesions. Clear or red lesions are more common in adolescents (**Figs. 1** and **2**)

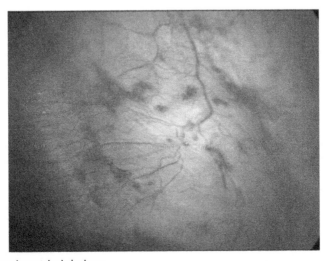

Fig. 1. Red endometriosis lesions.

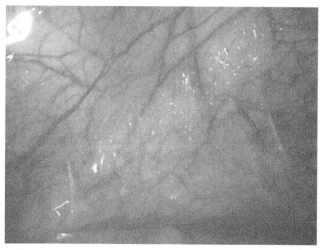

Fig. 2. Clear endometriosis lesions.

These atypical lesions have been shown to have active prostaglandin synthesis within them.[38] In 1 study of 20 adolescents with laparoscopically diagnosed endometriosis, 60% of the lesions seen at surgery were atypical red lesions. In the nonadolescent group in this same study, only 20% had red lesions.[39] Clear lesions can be more difficult to visualize; however, a technique has been described to aid in this visualization. The pelvis is filled with saline from the suction irrigator, and then the laparoscope is submerged in the fluid to minimize light reflection.[40] Because the positive predictive value for the visual detection of endometriosis is low (45%), it is important for all abnormal areas to be biopsied.[34]

The majority of adolescents with laparoscopically proven endometriosis have either stage 1 (77%–92%) or stage 2 (8%–23%) disease.[36,41] Common sights of endometriotic implants include the uterosacral ligaments, the posterior cul de sac, the pelvic sidewalls, and the ovaries.[39] During diagnostic laparoscopy, a systematic approach to the evaluation of the pelvis is necessary to improve the accuracy of surgical findings.

The treatment of endometriosis in adolescents is multidimensional; however, laparoscopy does play a role in those not responsive to medical management. Medical treatment induces atrophy of the hormonally dependent, ectopic endometrium, whereas surgical therapy aims to permanently destroy or remove the tissue. Patients younger than 18 years with persistent pelvic pain while taking combination hormone therapy should be offered a laparoscopic procedure for diagnosis and surgical management. The goal of therapy for adolescent endometriosis should be suppression of pain, suppression of disease progression, and preservation of fertility.[35] Repetitive surgical therapy is not advocated for adolescents because multiple surgeries can lead to adhesion formation and decreased fertility. In 1 study, 10% of adolescent patients underwent a second laparoscopy because of pelvic pain within 2 years of the index surgery.[39]

There are multiple ways to remove endometriotic implants, including laser ablation, electrocautery, and excision. One study compared coagulation with use of bipolar forceps and excision using laparoscopic scissors for superficial implants. Both treatment methods resulted in a low number of endometriosis-related symptoms after operative intervention. The coagulation group had a lower postoperative pain score at follow-up.[42] Excision, however, allows the benefit of a histologic specimen. Excision is performed by grasping the peritoneum with the endometriotic lesion to distance it from the underlying tissue. Laparoscopic scissors are used to remove the lesion along with a border of normal peritoneum. Surgical excision of endometriosis is reported to have a positive effect on dysmenorrhea and pelvic pain symptoms along with quality-of-life scores in adolescents.[39] Coagulation of implants spares deeper portions of disease from treatment and would not be beneficial for infiltrating disease.[32]

A recent study revealed that combined medical–laparoscopic surgical management prevents further stage progression of endometriotic disease in the adolescent population. Medical suppression of endometriotic implants can be achieved by cyclic or continuous combined oral contraceptive pills, depomedroxyprogesterone acetate, gonadotropin-releasing hormone agonists, or a levonorgestrel intrauterine device. The positive effect of combined medical–surgical treatment was determined by reviewing records of patients with biopsy-proven endometriosis treated with laparoscopic ablation and hormonal suppression, who underwent a second look laparoscopy. The median interval between surgeries was 29 months. No change in stage was observed among 70% of patients, 19% improved by a single stage, 1% improved by 2 stages, and 10% worsened by 1 stage.[43] A clear benefit of 1 medical therapy alone over another for treating endometriosis has not been shown, but this latter study clearly demonstrates the importance of multimodal approach to suppress disease.

Sequential laparoscopy in patients with endometriosis has shown that disease tends to become more severe without treatment. This is further illustrated by a recent case series of 3 adolescents (age 13–16) who were not compliant with postoperative medical suppression after initial laparoscopic coagulation of endometriotic lesions. On repeat laparoscopy owing to continued pain, 2 patients progressed from stage 1 to stage 4 over 2 years, whereas the other patient progressed from stage 1 to stage 2 over 5 years.[44]

Endometriosis can be a progressive, debilitating disease in the older pediatric patient. Prompt evaluation and treatment are necessary to prevent chronic pain and preserve fertility. Laparoscopy plays a vital role in diagnosis and treatment in those not responsive to medical management and is part of the multimodal approach to treating this population.

Adnexal Masses

Ovarian surgery during childhood can compromise future fertility because of the removal of normal ovarian tissue. Conservative surgery should be employed therefore to preserve ovarian tissue and minimize adhesion formation, and prevent recurrence of pathology.[45,46] Small, simple cysts (<2 cm) should be considered normal. The presence of enlarging, symptomatic, hormonally active ovarian cysts or those that show signs of malignancy should prompt operative intervention.[32] Adnexal masses without signs of malignancy on imaging or serum studies, can be treated laparoscopically.[46]

One study noted that gynecologists performed 79.9% of surgeries for ovarian masses in girls.[47] Laparoscopy is accepted as the gold standard in the management of adnexal masses in gynecology surgery, because it is associated with less postoperative discomfort and decreased hospital stay.[45,46] Laparoscopy for benign adnexal masses focuses on cystectomy, with preservation of the remainder of the ovary to maintain ovarian function. The stripping enucleation technique is a tissue-sparing procedure that is a favored approach to the benign adnexal mass[45] (**Fig. 3**). The ovarian cortex is incised using an energy source until the cyst wall is encountered.

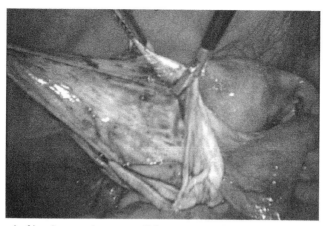

Fig. 3. Removal of benign ovarian cyst wall from surrounding ovarian cortex.

The cortex is then stripped away from the underlying cyst. This can be performed by either sharp, blunt, or aqua dissection.[32] With the latter, the suction irrigator is placed between the cortex and cyst wall and fluid is used to dissect the underlying cyst from the ovary.

Giant ovarian cysts can be ruptured upon trocar insertion during laparoscopy, and may also impede working space in the abdomen. A method has been described to puncture the cyst under direct visualization with the laparoscope. After puncture, the cystic fluid is removed with the suction irrigator. Once the cyst has been decompressed, there is more room in the pelvis to remove the cyst wall by enucleation.[32,45] Ultrasound-guided puncture followed by laparoscopic resection has also been described.[48]

One study identified variables associated with ovarian-conserving surgery in adolescents undergoing surgery for an adnexal mass. Of 82 patients under age 18, nongynecologic surgeons performed 35% of the surgeries, and gynecologists performed 65%. Gynecologists were significantly more likely to utilize laparoscopy than other surgeons (45% vs 13%, respectively). The presence of a gynecologic surgeon was also a highly significant predictor of ovarian-conserving surgery. Gynecologists conserved a portion of the ovary in 62% of cases compared with other surgeons in just 21% of cases.[49]

Because of the low frequency of malignant neoplasms in ovarian masses in children and adolescents, the laparoscopic resection of ovarian cysts is a safe operative approach that offers good cosmetic results, and focuses on preserving ovarian function.

Ovarian Torsion

Adnexal torsion is a gynecologic emergency as the vitality of the ovary and fallopian tube can be compromised if surgery is delayed. Torsion accounts for approximately 3% of all emergent gynecologic surgery.[50] As with adnexal masses, laparoscopy is used to manage ovarian torsion.

Torsion is most commonly associated with adnexal pathology, such as benign cystic teratomas, follicular cysts, tubal cysts, or serous or mucinous cystadenomas.[50] Paratubal cysts can also rarely undergo torsion involving the infundibulopelvic ligament and affect the ovary; however, torsion of a paratubal cyst involving the

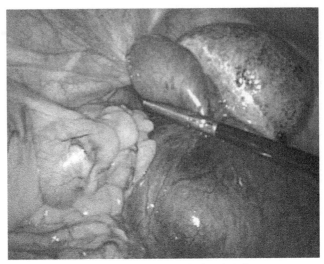

Fig. 4. Torsion of left adnexa involving the infundibulopelvic ligament.

uteroovarian ligament has also been reported[51] (**Fig. 4**). Fallopian tube torsion has also been described.[52] Malignant lesions are not commonly seen in torsion, because it is thought that malignancies may cause more inflammation and fibrosis leading to adhesive disease of surrounding structures.[47]

In the past, oophorectomy was the treatment of choice for a case of ovarian torsion. The rationale behind performing oophorectomy was the result of fear of risk of malignancy of the torsed ovary and the possible risk of thrombus into the systemic circulation after untwisting the affected adnexa. The risk of embolism after detorsion has now been widely negated.[53,54] Similarly, the risk of ovarian malignancy presenting as torsion is low. When there is no tumor seen at the time of surgery, the ovary can be left in place, or biopsies can be performed if the ovary seems to be suspicious for malignancy.[53]

When a conservative laparoscopic approach is performed, and the ovary is untwisted and left in situ, a follow-up ultrasound in 6 weeks can exclude a persistent cyst or tumor. Persistence or recurrence of cyst with normal tumor markers can be treated with laparoscopic ovarian cystectomy.[55] Detorsion can be safe and beneficial to ovarian function; it has been shown that even initially blue-to-black–appearing ovaries intraoperatively can subsequently have viable ovarian tissue and function.[50,56] Venous obstruction and stasis causes the adnexa to become dark and edematous, but most likely complete arterial obstruction has not occurred.[56] One study of 102 patients undergoing laparoscopic detorsion confirmed normal follicular development on the affected ovary on a 6-week postoperative ultrasonography. In patients who required subsequent surgery, the adnexa appeared normal in 13 out of 14 patients.[53] Another study of 40 patients ages 22 months to 17 years reported oophorectomy in 11 patients whose ovaries remained black–blue after initial detorsion. In 7 of the 11 patients, viable ovarian parenchyma was found in the surgical specimen.[55]

The risk of recurrence is low when adnexal torsion results from a mass and is treated with cystectomy. However, girls with torsion of normal adnexa treated conservatively may be at increased risk for future episodes. The management of recurrent torsion of normal adnexa remains controversial with regard to whether oopheropexy should be performed and whether one or both ovaries should be fixed.[57] Although ovarian torsion can have serious sequelae, such as recurrent torsion and potential loss of reproductive ovarian function, oopheropexy can also endanger the reproductive system by possibly interfering with blood supply, tubal function, or tubo-ovarian communication.[58,59]

Several techniques for performing oophoropexy have been discussed, including laparoscopic fixation of the ovary to the posterior abdominal wall, pelvic sidewall, or posterior uterus using nonabsorbable sutures, and plication of the utero-ovarian ligaments.[56,57,60,61] Fixing the ovary to the pelvic sidewall has been described using permanent suture from the mesovarium to the level of the pelvic brim. An incision can also be made into the ovary and titanium surgical clips used to plicate the ovary itself to the pelvic sidewall peritoneum.[60] Shortening of the utero-ovarian ligament has been argued by some to have less effect on future fertility because tubo-ovarian communication is not disrupted.[61] It is performed when a patient has an elongated uteroovarian ligament. This can be performed by suturing the proximal and distal ends of the ligament. Another option is to shorten the uteroovarian ligament by placement of an Endoloop in the midsection of the ligament.[60,61] The difficulty regarding the latter procedure is placement so that it is tight enough to not slip, but not too tight to cause tissue necrosis.[61]

One study of 102 patients with ovarian torsion had 12 patients with recurrent torsion, 7 of whom had recurrent torsion of normal adnexa. Unilateral oophoroxpexy was performed on 8 patients with recurrent torsion by different techniques and all patients undergoing oophoropexy had normal findings on follow-up ultrasonography.[57] This study argues that fixing only the involved adnexa seems to be adequate.

Children who have suffered from ovarian torsion may be increased risk of a repetitive event, either of the same ovary or contralateral ovary. In these recurrent cases, oophoropexy should be considered. The theoretical risk of interfering with tubal blood supply or function should be discussed with the patient and parents. Laparoscopy has allowed laparoscopic detorsion and oophoropexy to become minors procedure that can be performed in both children and adolescents. A conservative approach to blue–black ovaries after detorsion is safe and effective, and decreases unnecessary oophorectomies.

Ovarian Preservation in Children Undergoing Radiation

Laparoscopic oophoropexy is also used during the treatment of childhood cancers to help preserve fertility. Improved survival rates for childhood cancers have increased the demand for effective techniques to preserve fertility when gonadotoxic therapies are required. A minimally invasive approach to the procedure is safe and effective and allows adjuvant therapy to begin earlier compared with an approach by laparotomy. With laparoscopy, irradiation can be initiated within 1 week of oophoropexy. It has long been known that therapeutic radiation involving the pelvis is damaging to the ovaries. The effect of radiation on the ovary is age and dose dependent. Irreversible ovarian failure is certain at doses of 4 to 7 Gy in women older than 40 years of age. However, the ovaries are more resistant in prepubertal girls, and ovarian failure is not certain.[62]

The most common clinical scenarios presenting with ovarian preservation concerns are young girls with hematologic cancers or brain malignancies. In a study of 16 girls with acute lymphocytic leukemia undergoing total body irradiation, 56% had spontaneous puberty, but the remaining 7 subjects had ovarian failure.[63] Similarly primary ovarian damage has been reported to occur in more than 60% of girls receiving craniospinal radiation with or without chemotherapy for a brain tumor.[62]

In one 10-year follow-up study, oophoropexy was demonstrated to protect against radiation-induced ovarian failure in girls receiving spinal radiation. Oophoropexy was offered to girls 18 years of age or younger who were to undergo spinal radiation owing to brain malignancy. The most mobile ovary was selected for transposition. The infundibulopelvic ligament was skeletonized to allow the ovary to be moved to the lowest point in the pelvis and nonabsorbable silk sutures were used to attach the ovary to the uterosacral ligaments. Finally, the transposed and nontransposed ovaries were marked with titanium clips to aid in localization on radiation planning films. All patients underwent both spinal radiation therapy and chemotherapy. Overall, 13 of 15 patients in the oophoropexy group underwent puberty, and 2 (13%) showed signs of ovarian failure. In comparison, 5 of 11 (45%) in the nonoophoropexy group had evidence of ovarian dysfunction.[62]

These authors further argued use of a unilateral technique because if both ovaries are transposed there was concern that the patient would be committed to assisted reproductive therapy to achieve conception. With the unilateral technique, assisted reproductive therapy may be required if only the pexed ovary remains functional.[62]

One case reported laparoscopic medial oophoropexy performed 1 week before irradiation treatment for Hodgkin's lymphoma. Both ovaries were secured behind the uterus and the peritoneum lateral and parallel to each infundibulopelvic ligament was incised away from the lateral pelvic sidewalls to eliminate tension. The ovaries were transfixed to the posterior wall of the uterus using permanent suture. The patient began having spontaneous menses 16 months after completion of radiation and all gonadotropin levels remained normal. This case argues for medial oophoropexy as opposed to high lateral fixation of the ovaries, which requires transection of the uterine-ovarian ligament, disrupting a portion of the ovarian blood supply.[64]

Pregnancies in patients undergoing oophoropexy before radiation have been reported. One study evaluated 11 patients with a mean age of 13 who underwent bilateral ovarian transposition behind the uterus from 1972 to 1988 owing to Hodgkin's lymphoma. Fourteen pregnancies were recorded among these 11 women (12 live births and 3 miscarriages). None of the women needed the ovaries to be relocated and none needed assisted reproductive therapy.[65]

Mullerian Anomalies

Congenital malformations of the female genital tract result from the disturbance of either formation or fusion of the Mullerian ducts. A unicornuate uterus covers a wide range of anomalies and may exist alone or more commonly with rudimentary noncommunicating horn, estimated to be present 75% to 90% of the time. The prevalence of this type of uterine malformation has been reported to range between 2.4% and 13.7% of all cases of uterine anomalies.[66] This diagnosis may be suspected in any female with a history of cyclical pelvic pain even in the absence of monthly menses.[67] Removal of the rudimentary horn and its ipsilateral tube upon diagnosis as early as the adolescent age is recommended, to relieve the symptoms of dysmenorrhea and to avoid serious future complications such as endometriosis, ectopic pregnancy, and uterine horn rupture. In recent years, laparoscopy has become a viable alternative to laparotomy for the management of uterine congenital anomalies.[68]

The majority of girls with mullerian anomalies are asymptomatic and therefore do not require treatment. However, some women may present with symptoms owing to an obstructed system, such as abdominal pain and dysmenorrhea. The most common time to present with symptoms of an obstructed horn is in the teenage years. An intravenous urogram should be performed to assess the course and number of the

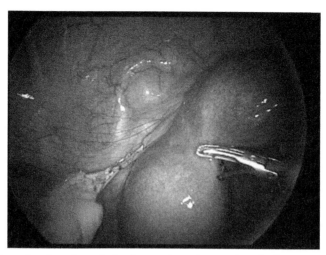

Fig. 5. Excision of rudimentary uterine horn using a harmonic scalpel.

ureters, as the incidence of renal tract anomalies varies from 31% to 100%. One review focused on 15 patients who underwent laparoscopic removal of a uterine horn. In each case, the ipsilateral ureter was identified in its position related to the uterus. Bladder integrity was also confirmed either by instilling methylene blue into the bladder or performing a cystoscopy at the end of the procedure. Seven patients had renal agenesis ipsilateral to the mullerian anomaly. In all cases, it was decided to remove the ipsilateral fallopian tube to avoid the risk of ectopic pregnancies, but the ipsilateral ovary was preserved.[69]

A noncommunicating uterine horn can be resected using the surgeon's vessel sealing technology of choice. The approach is comparable to performing a hysterectomy, because access to the retroperitoneum is obtained by dividing the round ligament. The anterior and posterior leaves of the broad ligament can then be separated to reveal the uterine vessels on the side of the horn. The avascular midline fibrous section between the 2 horns can be incised freeing the rudimentary horn (**Figs. 5** and **6**). Chromotubation can be performed to demonstrate patency of the normal uterus and display any evidence of any defect from the area incised. The use of the harmonic scalpel is has been described as an ideal instrument to use for such an adolescent case because it is minimally invasive and requires only a 5-mm port site. It can also be used to vaporize endometriotic lesions that can often be present.[67]

In a noncommunicating rudimentary horn, retrograde menstruation can occur, which leads to pelvic endometriosis. One case report describes giving 6 months of preoperative gonadotropin-releasing hormone agonist therapy to a patient before operative laparoscopy to decrease the amount of pelvic disease. The rudimentary horn was then able to be freed from adjacent structures and removed.[68] Retrograde menstruation from the rudimentary horn through the ipsilateral fallopian tube could result in the development of a hematosalpinx and endometriosis. Patients with unicornuate uterus are reported to have a significantly greater prevalence of endometriosis than other uterine anomalies. If severe endometriosis is suspected, the use of a gonadotropin-releasing hormone analog would reduce vascularity and facilitate surgery.[69]

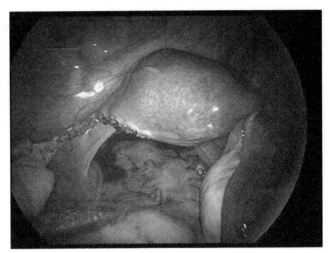

Fig. 6. Remaining unicornuate uterus after excisions of rudimentary uterine horn.

There is good correlation between magnetic resonance imaging and operative findings, especially with uterine structure.[70] Renal anomalies can also be identified. The laparoscopic technique is associated with a shortened hospital stay and improved cosmesis, along with a quicker return to normal activity.

Single-Incision Laparoscopy

To date, there has been very little written about the use of single incision laparoscopic surgery (SILS) in the pediatric population. SILS utilizes a single umbilical incision, with or without a specialized port. Considering the small body surface of children, there are possible benefits of reducing the number of incisions; however, many abdominal operations can be done with a 5-mm umbilical port and stab incisions for 2.7-mm instruments placed directly through the abdominal wall. These incisions typically leave no perceptible scarring.[71] There is evidence to suggest that visible scarring on the face and neck in children can result in reduced self-esteem, impaired socialization skills, and lower self-ratings of problem-solving ability. It is not clear whether abdominal scarring has the same magnitude of negative effects, because such scars are usually not visible.[72]

Cases reported using SILS in children include cholecystectomy, appendectomy, enterolysis, ovarian cystectomy, and hernia repair.[71-73] In a study of 20 pediatric patients at Stanford undergoing various pediatric surgeries using SILS, there were no conversions to standard laparoscopy or an open operation. Intravenous analgesia requirements and hospital length of stay mirrored that of standard laparoscopy and all families were pleased with the cosmetic result.[72]

Trocars are placed through a single incision in a triangular configuration. This parallel co-location of the instruments can sometimes lead to instrument collisions and difficult angles of resection. One study looked at placing the operating scope through an umbilical incision and placing a separate 3-mm port in another location depending upon the procedure. The addition of a single 3-mm instrument at a separate site allows for easier dissection and triangulation, with almost no visible scarring. This study attempted to evaluate the single port technique, but acknowledged the inherent differences in children's' body surface area and demonstrated that the addition of 1 small port can give similar outcomes.[73]

The clear benefits of eliminating 1-, 2-, 3-, 5-, or even 10-mm ports in favor of a 15- to 20-mm umbilical incision has not been clearly demonstrated. There is also concern that the larger umbilical incision may be associated with more pain and risk of developing an incisional hernia. The current single incision multiports require at least a 20-mm incision, which is larger than the umbilicus in virtually all small children. This is thought to devalue the proposed cosmetic benefit.[71,72] More experience is needed to assess whether there is a benefit over standard laparoscopy in the pediatric population.

SUMMARY

Minimally invasive surgery is now standard of care for many procedures in pediatric gynecology. Laparoscopy has been well documented to produce faster recovery, decreased postoperative pain, and because of smaller incisions, a better cosmetic result. These are important when considering an active pediatric patient. Although a laparoscopic approach to endometriosis, adnexal masses, and ovarian torsion are well supported in the literature in the pediatric patient, more data are needed with regard to SILS in younger patients. Laparoscopy seems to be a better approach to oopheropexy in children undergoing radiation, and in resection of certain mullerian anomalies; however, the numbers are low.

Similarly in pregnant patients, laparoscopy provides for shorter recovery times, decrease analgesic use and shorter hospital stays. Concerns about poor fetal outcomes in surgery during pregnancy for non gynecologic problems have been brought to light; however, the evidence indicates that these outcomes can be attributed to the nature of the underlying disease and not the surgical approach. With regard to pneumoperitoneum the effect of CO_2 insufflation on fetal physiology and long-term outcomes remains unclear, and will continue to be an issue of controversy until larger studies are published.

With both the pediatric and pregnant populations, laparoscopic complications can be diminished when performed by skilled surgeons with strict adherence to good technical principles. The advantages of laparoscopy are great, and this approach should be considered in pediatric and pregnant patients.

REFERENCES

1. Nezhat F, Nezhat C, Silfen SL, et al. Laparoscopic ovarian cystectomy during pregnancy. J Laparoendosc Surg 1991;1:161–4.
2. Halkic N, Tempia-Caliera AA, Ksontini R, et al. Laparoscopic management of appendicitis and symptomatic cholelithiasis during pregnancy. Langenbecks Arch Surg 2006;391:467–71.
3. Sadot E, Telem DA, Arora M, et al. Laparoscopy: a safe approach to appendicitis during pregnancy. Surg Endosc 2010;24:383–9.
4. Buser KB. Laparoscopic surgery in the pregnant patient: results and recommendations. JSLS 2009;13:32–5.
5. Patel SG, Veverka TJ. Laparoscopic cholecystectomy in pregnancy. Curr Surg 2002;59:74–8.
6. Jackson H, Granger S, Price R, et al. Diagnosis and laparoscopic treatment of surgical diseases during pregnancy: an evidence-based review. Surg Endosc 2008;22:1917–27.
7. Fatum M, Rojansky N. Laparoscopic surgery during pregnancy. Obstet Gynecol Surv 2001;56:50–9.

8. Roman H, Accoceberry M, Bolandard F, et al. Laparoscopic management of a ruptured benign dermoid cyst during advanced pregnancy. J Minim Invasive Gynecol 2005;12:377–8.

9. Patacchiola F, Collevecchio N, Di Ferdinando A, et al. Management of ovarian cysts in pregnancy: a case report. Eur J Gynaecol Oncol 2005;26:651–3.

10. Johnson JR, Lee C, Carnett S, et al. Laparoscopic management of enlarged serous cystadenoma in advanced pregnancy. J Minim Invasive Gynecol 2007;14:247–9.

11. Sturlese E, Retto G, Pulia A, et al. Laparoscopic salpingo-oophorectomy during pregnancy: a case report. Clin Exp Obstet Gynecol 2000;27:61–2.

12. Stepp KJ, Tulikangas PK, Goldberg JM, et al. Laparoscopy for adnexal masses in the second trimester of pregnancy. J Am Assoc Gynecol Laparosc 2003;10:55–9.

13. Bassil S, Steinhart U, Donnez J. Successful laparoscopic management of adnexal torsion during week 25 of a twin pregnancy. Hum Reprod 1999;14:855–7.

14. Soriano D, Yefet Y, Seidman DS, et al. Laparoscopy versus laparotomy in the management of adnexal masses during pregnancy. Fertil Steril 1999;71:955–60.

15. Yuen PM, Ng PS, Leung PL, et al. Outcome in laparoscopic management of persistent adnexal mass during the second trimester of pregnancy. Surg Endosc 2004;18:1354–7.

16. Conron RW Jr, Abbruzzi K, Cochrane SO, et al. Laparoscopic procedures in pregnancy. Am Surg 1999;65:259–63.

17. Moore RD, Smith WG. Laparoscopic management of adnexal masses in pregnant women. J Reprod Med 1999;44:97–100.

18. Thomas SJ, Brisson P. Laparoscopic appendectomy and cholecystectomy during pregnancy: six case reports. JSLS 1998;2:41–6.

19. Carter JF, Soper DE. Operative laparoscopy in pregnancy. JSLS 2004;8:57–60.

20. Shay DC, Bhavani-Shankar K, Datta S. Laparoscopic surgery during pregnancy. Anesthesiol Clin North Am 2001;19:57–67.

21. O'Rourke N, Kodali BS. Laparoscopic surgery during pregnancy. Curr Opin Anaesthesiol 2006;19:254–9.

22. Chohan L, Kilpatrick CC. Laparoscopy in pregnancy: a literature review. Clin Obstet Gynecol 2009;52:557–69.

23. Bhavani-Shankar K, Steinbrook RA, Brooks DC, et al. Arterial to end-tidal carbon dioxide pressure difference during laparoscopic surgery in pregnancy. Anesthesiology 2000;93:370–3.

24. Rollins MD, Chan KJ, Price RR. Laparoscopy for appendicitis and cholelithiasis during pregnancy: a new standard of care. Surg Endosc 2004;18:237–41.

25. Lachman E, Schienfeld A, Voss E, et al. Pregnancy and laparoscopic surgery. J Am Assoc Gynecol Laparosc 1999;6:347–51.

26. Akira S, Yamanaka A, Ishihara T, et al. Gasless laparoscopic ovarian cystectomy during pregnancy: comparison with laparotomy. Am J Obstet Gynecol 1999;180:554–7.

27. Tanaka H, Futamura N, Takubo S, et al. Gasless laparoscopy under epidural anesthesia for adnexal cysts during pregnancy. J Reprod Med 1999;44:929–32.

28. Yumi H. Guidelines for diagnosis, treatment, and use of laparoscopy for surgical problems during pregnancy: this statement was reviewed and approved by the Board of Governors of the Society of American Gastrointestinal and Endoscopic Surgeons (SAGES), September 2007. It was prepared by the SAGES Guidelines Committee. Surg Endosc 2008;22:849–61.

29. Rizzo AG. Laparoscopic surgery in pregnancy: long-term follow-up. J Laparoendosc Adv Surg Tech A 2003;13:11–5.

30. Amos JD, Schorr SJ, Norman PF, et al. Laparoscopic surgery during pregnancy. Am J Surg 1996;171:435–7.
31. Reynolds JD, Booth JV, de la Fuente S, et al. A review of laparoscopy for non-obstetric-related surgery during pregnancy. Curr Surg 2003;60:164–73.
32. Broach AN, Mansuria SM, Sanfilippo JS. Pediatric and adolescent gynecologic laparoscopy. Clin Obstet Gynecol 2009;52:380–9.
33. Ahmad G, Duffy JM, Phillips K, et al. Laparoscopic entry techniques. Cochrane Database Syst Rev 2008:CD006583.
34. Attaran M, Gidwani GP. Adolescent endometriosis. Obstet Gynecol Clin North Am 2003;30:379–90.
35. American College of Obstetricians and Gynecologists. ACOG committee opinion. Number 310, April 2005. Endometriosis in adolescents. Obstet Gynecol 2005;105:921–7.
36. Laufer MR, Goitein L, Bush M, et al. Prevalence of endometriosis in adolescent girls with chronic pelvic pain not responding to conventional therapy. J Pediatr Adolesc Gynecol 1997;10:199–202.
37. Simpson JL, Elias S, Malinak LR, et al. Heritable aspects of endometriosis. I. Genetic studies. Am J Obstet Gynecol 1980;137:327–31.
38. Dovey S, Sanfilippo J. Endometriosis and the adolescent. Clin Obstet Gynecol 2010;53:420–8.
39. Roman JD. Adolescent endometriosis in the Waikato region of New Zealand: a comparative cohort study with a mean follow-up time of 2.6 years. Aust N Z J Obstet Gynaecol 2010;50:179–83.
40. Laufer MR. Identification of clear vesicular lesions of atypical endometriosis: a new technique. Fertil Steril 1997;68:739–40.
41. Emmert C, Romann D, Riedel HH. Endometriosis diagnosed by laparoscopy in adolescent girls. Arch Gynecol Obstet 1998;261:89–93.
42. Radosa MP, Bernardi TS, Georgiev I, et al. Coagulation versus excision of primary superficial endometriosis: a 2-year follow-up. Eur J Obstet Gynecol Reprod Biol 2010;150:195–8.
43. Doyle JO, Missmer SA, Laufer MR. The effect of combined surgical-medical intervention on the progression of endometriosis in an adolescent and young adult population. J Pediatr Adolesc Gynecol 2009;22:257–63.
44. Unger CA, Laufer MR. Progression of endometriosis in non-medically managed adolescents: a case series. J Pediatr Adolesc Gynecol 2011;24:e21–3.
45. Mayer JP, Bettolli M, Kolberg-Schwerdt A, et al. Laparoscopic approach to ovarian mass in children and adolescents: already a standard in therapy. J Laparoendosc Adv Surg Tech A 2009;19(Suppl 1):S111–5.
46. Deligeoroglou E, Eleftheriades M, Shiadoes V, et al. Ovarian masses during adolescence: clinical, ultrasonographic and pathologic findings, serum tumor markers and endocrinological profile. Gynecol Endocrinol 2004;19:1–8.
47. Templeman C, Fallat ME, Blinchevsky A, et al. Noninflammatory ovarian masses in girls and young women. Obstet Gynecol 2000;96:229–33.
48. Ates O, Karakaya E, Hakguder G, et al. Laparoscopic excision of a giant ovarian cyst after ultrasound-guided drainage. J Pediatr Surg 2006;41:E9–11.
49. Bristow RE, Nugent AC, Zahurak ML, et al. Impact of surgeon specialty on ovarian-conserving surgery in young females with an adnexal mass. J Adolesc Health 2006;39:411–6.
50. Breech LL, Hillard PJ. Adnexal torsion in pediatric and adolescent girls. Curr Opin Obstet Gynecol 2005;17:483–9.

51. Dietrich JE, Heard MJ, Edwards C. Uteroovarian ligament torsion of the due to a paratubal cyst. J Pediatr Adolesc Gynecol 2005;18:125–7.
52. Antoniou N, Varras M, Akrivis C, et al. Isolated torsion of the fallopian tube: a case report and review of the literature. Clin Exp Obstet Gynecol 2004;31:235–8.
53. Oelsner G, Cohen SB, Soriano D, et al. Minimal surgery for the twisted ischaemic adnexa can preserve ovarian function. Hum Reprod 2003;18:2599–602.
54. McGovern PG, Noah R, Koenigsberg R, et al. Adnexal torsion and pulmonary embolism: case report and review of the literature. Obstet Gynecol Surv 1999;54:601–8.
55. Galinier P, Carfagna L, Delsol M, et al. Ovarian torsion. Management and ovarian prognosis: a report of 45 cases. J Pediatr Surg 2009;44:1759–65.
56. Celik A, Ergun O, Aldemir H, et al. Long-term results of conservative management of adnexal torsion in children. J Pediatr Surg 2005;40:704–8.
57. Fuchs N, Smorgick N, Tovbin Y, et al. Oophoropexy to prevent adnexal torsion: how, when, and for whom? J Minim Invasive Gynecol 2010;17:205–8.
58. Pansky M, Smorgick N, Herman A, et al. Torsion of normal adnexa in postmenarchal women and risk of recurrence. Obstet Gynecol 2007;109:355–9.
59. Crouch NS, Gyampoh B, Cutner AS, et al. Ovarian torsion: to pex or not to pex? Case report and review of the literature. J Pediatr Adolesc Gynecol 2003;16:381–4.
60. Rollene N, Nunn M, Wilson T, et al. Recurrent ovarian torsion in a premenarchal adolescent girl: contemporary surgical management. Obstet Gynecol 2009;114: 422–4.
61. Weitzman VN, DiLuigi AJ, Maier DB, et al. Prevention of recurrent adnexal torsion. Fertil Steril 2008;90:2018.
62. Kuohung W, Ram K, Cheng DM, et al. Laparoscopic oophoropexy prior to radiation for pediatric brain tumor and subsequent ovarian function. Hum Reprod 2008;23: 117–21.
63. Sarafoglou K, Boulad F, Gillio A, et al. Gonadal function after bone marrow transplantation for acute leukemia during childhood. J Pediatr 1997;130:210–6.
64. Scott SM, Schlaff W. Laparoscopic medial oophoropexy prior to radiation therapy in an adolescent with Hodgkin's disease. J Pediatr Adolesc Gynecol 2005;18:355–7.
65. Terenziani M, Piva L, Meazza C, et al. Oophoropexy: a relevant role in preservation of ovarian function after pelvic irradiation. Fertil Steril 2009;91:935 e15–6.
66. American Fertility Society. The American Fertility Society classifications of adnexal adhesions, distal tubal occlusion, tubal occlusion secondary to tubal ligation, tubal pregnancies, mullerian anomalies and intrauterine adhesions. Fertil Steril 1988;49:944–55.
67. Dietrich JE, Young AE, Young RL. Resection of a non-communicating uterine horn with use of the harmonic scalpel. J Pediatr Adolesc Gynecol 2004;17:407–9.
68. Liatsikos SA, Tsikouras P, Souftas V, et al. Diagnosis and laparoscopic management of a rudimentary uterine horn in a teenage girl, presenting with haematometra and severe endometriosis: our experience and review of literature. Minim Invasive Ther Allied Technol 2010;19:241–7.
69. Strawbridge LC, Crouch NS, Cutner AS, et al. Obstructive mullerian anomalies and modern laparoscopic managoment. J Pediatr Adolesc Gynecol 2007;20:195–200.
70. Minto CL, Hollings N, Hall-Craggs M, et al. Magnetic resonance imaging in the assessment of complex Mullerian anomalies. BJOG 2001;108:791–7.
71. Garey CL, Laituri CA, Ostlie DJ, et al. A review of single site minimally invasive surgery in infants and children. Pediatr Surg Int 2010;26:451–6.
72. Dutta S. Early experience with single incision laparoscopic surgery: eliminating the scar from abdominal operations. J Pediatr Surg 2009;44:1741–5.
73. Rothenberg SS, Shipman K, Yoder S Experience with modified single-port laparoscopic procedures in children. J Laparoendosc Adv Surg Tech A 2009;19:695–8.

The Core of a Competent Surgeon: A Working Knowledge of Surgical Anatomy and Safe Dissection Techniques

Robert M. Rogers Jr, MD, Richard H. Taylor, MD

KEYWORDS
- Anatomy • Dissection • Surgical skills • Technique

The core skills of a competent surgeon are hands-on knowledge of relevant surgical anatomy and the safe exposure of that anatomy. Although the surgeon knows the area of the pelvis in which he or she is operating and the structural anatomy contained therein, the surgeon must skillfully expose that anatomy to sight and/or palpation by expert dissection methods. These techniques of surgical dissection are universal to any competent surgeon in any surgical dissection field, using any instruments or mode of surgery, including laparoscopy and the daVinci system robot. This article discusses the specific dissection techniques of expert surgeons, the rationale for their use, and then defines the anatomic areas of gynecologic surgery in the pelvis and the relevant structural anatomy that defines each of these areas. No surgeon can expect surgical outcomes to be any better than their surgical dissection skills.

SURGICAL DISSECTION

The purpose of surgical dissection is to expose anatomic structures while safeguarding their structural and physiologic integrity. Also, the competent surgical dissector minimizes bleeding in the surgical field to fully visualize the tissues and anatomic structures relevant to his operation. The actual progression of dissection is a purposeful "millimeter by millimeter."

Portions of the text appeared previously in Rogers RM, Taylor RH. Surgical dissection and anatomy of the female pelvis for the gynecologic surgeon. In: Gomel V, Brill AI, eds. Reconstructive and Reproductive Surgery in Gynecology. New York and London: Informa Healthcare, 2010. The authors have nothing to disclose.
Northwest Women's Health Care, 75 Claremont Street, Suite A, Kalispell, MT 59901
* Corresponding author.
E-mail address: shirdoc@aol.com

Obstet Gynecol Clin N Am 38 (2011) 777–788
doi:10.1016/j.ogc.2011.10.003
0889-8545/11/$ – see front matter © 2011 Published by Elsevier Inc.

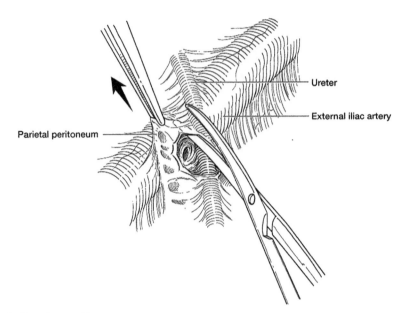

Ureter

External iliac artery

Parietal peritoneum

Fig. 1. Grasping peritoneum.

The purpose of these maneuvers is to thin out visceral connective tissues and any scarring so that the relevant structures can be clearly identified by sight and/or palpation. The surgeon must not cut, ligate, or coagulate any tissue is not seen or understood. Therefore, any surgical dissection, sharp and blunt, must proceed "millimeter by millimeter." The steps of dissection thin out connective tissues to reveal the structural anatomy embedded therein. The surgeon must be able to visualize these structures and their spatial orientation within the dissection field in his or her mind. Dissection must reveal the anatomy, not obscure the dissection field or confuse appearance. The surgeon uses the instruments, sight, and a learned ability to palpate to perform the surgical dissection. Knowledge of the structures contained within the particular field of dissection is as essential as the hands-on techniques. This also requires the operator in her or his mind to visualize in 3 dimensions.

By progressing "millimeter by millimeter" in the dissection, the operator achieves 4 goals. First, correct orientation and direction of dissection are maintained. Second, there is step-by-step control of instruments used and techniques employed. There is time to evaluate and change dissection techniques, direction of approach, and/or instrumentation used. Flexibility, ingenuity, and experience are essential characteristics of the accomplished surgeon. Third, therefore, the anatomic structures can be safely explored and dissected. Fourth, any injury to a viscus or blood vessel will be limited to 1 to 2 mm. By dissecting deliberately and slowly, in most cases the operator can readily control any bleeding encountered or see/feel an unavoidable injury to a viscus or structure. Therefore, significant bleeding or gross visceral injury should be minimized.

The techniques of expert surgical dissection are "grasp and tent," "millimeter" incision under direct visual control (**Fig. 1**), "push-spread" (**Fig. 2**), "traction-counter-traction" (**Fig. 3**), "gently wiping/teasing" of the tissues (**Fig. 4**), and hydrodissection. Hydrodissection is the injection of sterile fluid into the surgical field to tent and thin out the connective tissue fibers.

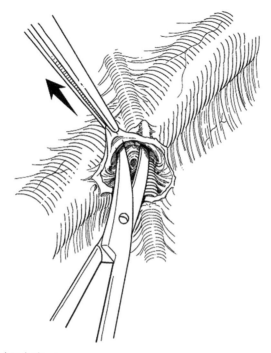

Fig. 2. Push-spread technique.

By "grasping and tenting" the peritoneum or tissue to be incised, the operator elevates the tissue away from a vital structure—ureter, artery, vein, bowel, bladder, and nerve. Grasping and tenting of the tissues also thins out the grasped tissue, so that an edge of bowel can be seen, for example. A millimeter incision can then be made without concern for underlying structures. With the gentle "push–spread" or "poke and open" technique, the operator further thins out the connective tissues and dense scarring to see what structures are present therein. This step is also aided by gentle traction and countertraction and further tenting before further cutting or gentle

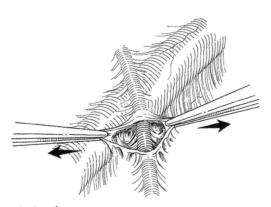

Fig. 3. Traction–countertraction.

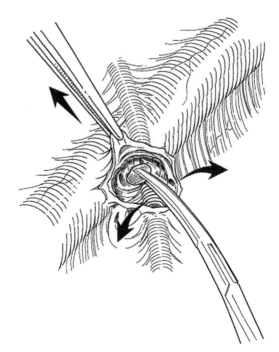

Fig. 4. Gently wiping/teasing of tissues.

"wiping" ensues. Dissection should proceed millimeter by millimeter from easy-to-dissect, known areas of anatomy to denser, more difficult areas of dissection. With experience, the operator will be conditioned to the sight and feel of the safe dissection techniques that can be used in each area of the pelvis. Wiping should also proceed gently, millimeter by millimeter, to further thin out the tissues. Broad blunt and quick stokes of wiping the tissues may result in uncontrolled entry into a viscus or tearing into a blood vessel. Wiping should progress gently.

The technique of hydrodissection can facilitate dissections in the pelvic sidewall and potential spaces, such as the retropubic space, vesicovaginal space, paravaginal and pararectal spaces, and rectovaginal space. Hydrodissection is especially useful in performing vaginal dissections in preparation for placement of sutures, graft material, and permanent meshes in reparative vaginal procedures.

When observing a competent surgeon performing surgery in the operating room or on a video, the student of surgery must focus and ask 2 key questions: "Where in the pelvis is the surgeon operating?" and "Which dissection techniques is the surgeon using?" The first question makes the learner think of the anatomy contained within that particular field of dissection. The second question makes the student appreciate and focus on learning the true skills of the competent surgeon. In using this pattern of asking directed questions, the less experienced surgeon can prepare his or her eyes to observe and his or her mind to concentrate for relevant learning—learning that can and will immediately improve the skills of tissue dissection used in the next surgical procedure. The student can only learn what the mind has been prepared to learn and what the eyes have been prepared to observe.

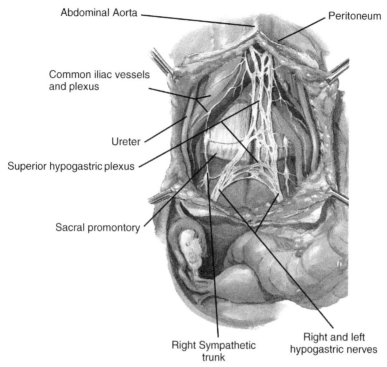

Abdominal Aorta

Peritoneum

Common iliac vessels and plexus

Ureter

Superior hypogastric plexus

Sacral promontory

Right Sympathetic trunk

Right and left hypogastric nerves

Fig. 5. Presacral space. (*From* Netter: Atlas of Human Anatomy, 5e. Elsevier 2010, plate 383, p. 392.): (Reprinted with permission from Netter Anatomy Illustration Collection, © Elsevier Inc. All Rights Reserved.)

PELVIC AREAS OF SURGICAL DISSECTION IN GYNECOLOGY

The specific areas of surgical dissection must be learned and visualized with much practice at the operating table, as well as by study and repetition. This knowledge is essential for the competent surgeon. The specific areas of surgical dissection within the female pelvis are the presacral space; the pelvic brim; the pelvic sidewall; the level of the cervicouterine junction where the ureter and uterine vessels cross; the paravesical/paravaginal area, leading to the retropubic space of Retzius; the vesico-vaginal space; and the pararectal space and rectovaginal space. These spaces may also be accessed via the vaginal route, as well as by laparotomy and laparoscopy.

"Presacral" Space

The "presacral" space (**Fig. 5**) is important to gynecologic surgeons when performing a "presacral" neurectomy, when removing presacral nodes, or when performing a sacral colpopexy for support of the prolapsed vaginal apex. "Presacral" is a misnomer because this surgical area is just in front of the fourth and fifth lumbar vertebrae. The correct terminology is the lower "prelumbar" space. This space is bounded anteriorly by the parietal peritoneum and posteriorly by the anterior longitudinal ligament over the lowest 2 lumbar vertebrae and the promontory of the sacrum. The middle sacral artery and a plexus of veins are attached superficial to the anterior longitudinal ligament. The visceral fascia in this space envelopes fatty areolar tissue, visceral

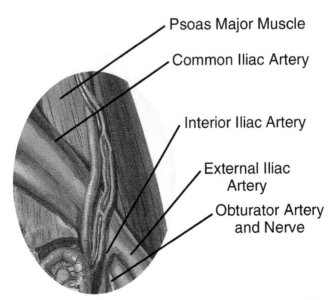

Psoas Major Muscle

Common Iliac Artery

Interior Iliac Artery

External Iliac
Artery

Obturator Artery
and Nerve

Fig. 6. Pelvic brim. (*From* Netter: Atlas of Human Anatomy, 5e. Elsevier 2010, plate 383, p. 392.): (Reprinted with permission from Netter Anatomy Illustration Collection, © Elsevier Inc. All Rights Reserved.)

nerves, and lymphatic tissue. There is no one "presacral," nerve but a multitude of finer visceral nerves that course through, or even around, this area over the common iliac vessels. The "presacral" nerves are the fibers of the superior hypogastric plexus which is located here.

The right lateral boundary of the "presacral" space is the right common iliac artery and the right ureter. The left lateral border is the left common iliac vein and left ureter, as well as the inferior mesenteric artery and vein traversing through the mesentery of the sigmoid colon. All of these structures must be identified when dissecting in this space. When performing a "presacral" neurectomy, the operator must excise all fatty areolar tissue in this area, because it contains the visceral nerves that need to be ablated. Because these nerves may not travel in the central portion of the space but may be more lateral toward the iliac arteries and veins, the surgeon must dissect as laterally as possible without injuring the vital structures along its borders. Lateral and inferior dissection in the "presacral" space leads to the structures entering the pelvis over the pelvic brim.

Pelvic Brim

The pelvic brim (**Fig. 6**) at the sacroiliac joint is a very important location for the entry of multiple structures into the pelvic cavity and must be appreciated layer by layer. From the peritoneal surface, working posteriorly to the sacroiliac juncture, the following structures are found crisscrossing over one another: The peritoneum, the ovarian vessels in the infundibulopelvic ligament, the ureter passing over the bifurcation of the common iliac artery, the common iliac vein, the medial edge of the psoas muscle, the obturator nerve, and the parietal fascia just over the capsule of the sacroiliac joint. Just medial to the obturator nerve not seen is the lumbosacral trunk of somatic nerves traveling from the lumbar plexus to the sacral plexus of nerves. Because of the proximity of the

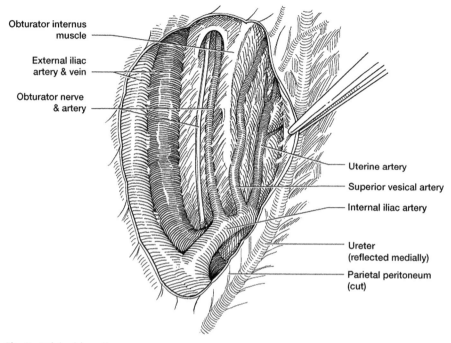

Obturator internus muscle

External iliac artery & vein

Obturator nerve & artery

Uterine artery

Superior vesical artery

Internal iliac artery

Ureter (reflected medially)

Parietal peritoneum (cut)

Fig. 7. Pelvic sidewall.

ovarian vessels over the ureter at this level, the laparoscopic operator must realize that ureteral injury can occur during ligation or coagulation of the infundibulopelvic ligament. These structures then enter the pelvis, rotate 90° and travel within the pelvic sidewall.

Pelvic Sidewall

Based on avascular planes, the pelvic sidewall (**Fig. 7**) consists of 3 surgical layers medial to lateral. The first layer is the parietal peritoneum with the attached ureter in its own endopelvic visceral fascial sheath. When this peritoneum is incised and retracted medially during the first operative procedure, the ureter comes with it.

The second surgical layer consists of the internal iliac (hypogastric) artery and vein and their visceral anterior tributaries, all enveloped within the endopelvic visceral fascia, which also envelopes the lymph tissue, the visceral nerves, and fat deposits. Blunt dissection easily separates the first surgical layer from the second surgical layer in an avascular manner. Contained within the second surgical layer are the visceral branches of the internal iliac artery (including the uterine), the superior vesical leading to the obliterated umbilical, the inferior vesical, the vaginal, and the middle rectal. During retroperitoneal sidewall dissection, retraction of the obliterated umbilical artery places the superior vesical artery on stretch, which points the operator to the internal iliac artery. Thus, this second sidewall layer can be readily located. The medial offshoot where the superior vesical artery enters the internal iliac artery is the uterine artery. This second surgical layer consist of visceral anatomic structures (visceral blood vessels, visceral nerves, and lymph vessels and nodes) that service the pelvic viscera—bladder, ureter, uterus and vagina, and rectum.

The internal pudendal, the inferior gluteal, and the obturator arteries are the parietal branches of the internal iliac and promptly course into or along parietal fascia. During dissection in this second surgical layer, any of these arteries and veins may be occluded for the purposes of hemostasis without any adverse reactions. The rich collateral blood circulation in the pelvis permits this. However, to emphasize, the operator must not perform any procedures in this second surgical layer until the ureter (first surgical layer), the external iliac vessels, and obturator nerve and vessels (third surgical layer) have been positively identified. The laparoscopic surgeon must take great care in avoiding any laceration or injury to the ureter, external iliac vessels, or obturator nerve.

The third surgical layer of the pelvic sidewall consists of 2 elements: The external iliac artery and vein on the medial aspect of the psoas muscle, and the parietal fascia over the obturator internus muscle, with the obturator nerve, artery, and vein allowed to remain along this muscle, although the obturator nerve may at times be retracted medially. Likewise, blunt dissection along the obturator internus fascia easily allows the second surgical layer of visceral arteries and veins to be retracted medially in an avascular manner. This is accomplished in dissections in the paravesical/paravaginal space. In fact, this may be done down to the level of the ischial spine, where the obturator internus muscle tendon exits the pelvis through the lesser sciatic foramen. This knowledge is important in performing laparoscopic paravaginal defect repairs. During paravaginal repairs, this area is approached through the retropubic space of Retzius.

In another perspective from anterior to posterior, the pelvic sidewall may be easily viewed through the laparoscope through the peritoneal covering, especially on the right side. Anteriorly is found the psoas muscle. On its medial aspect is the external iliac artery with the external iliac vein just medial and posterior to it. Just underneath the external iliac vein is the bony ridge of the arcuate line of the ilium, which cannot be seen. Also not seen are the obturator nerve, artery, and vein coursing underneath this ridge along the anterior border of the obturator internus muscle, traveling toward the obturator canal, found on the underside of the superior pubic ramus. However, in the thinner patient, the ureter and the internal iliac artery are easily seen several centimeters below the external iliac vein, traveling in parallel in an almost horizontal position in the supine patient. The ureter characteristically peristalses, whereas the internal iliac artery, just posterior to the ureter, characteristically pulsates with the beating of the heart.

Level of the Cervicouterine Junction

The cardinal ligament at the base of the broad ligament is found at the level of the cervicouterine junction, and contains the uterine artery traveling medially toward the lower uterine segment. Dissection of the pelvic sidewall naturally leads into this area. The surgical area located next to the lower uterine segment is known as the parametrium. That area located just lateral to the vagina is called the upper paracolpium. The uterine artery branches medially from the internal iliac artery, whereas the more lateral terminal branch of the uterine artery continues as the superior vesical artery, and then into the obliterated umbilical artery. The origin of the uterine artery may be laparoscopically identified by dissecting along the medial border of the obliterated umbilical artery while working backward toward the internal iliac artery. The medial offshoot is then identified as the uterine artery.

Approximately 0.5 to 1 cm lateral to the cervicouterine junction, the uterine artery and vein trifurcate into the ascending, transverse, and descending uterine vessels. This information is important for ligation or coagulation/sealing of the vasculature

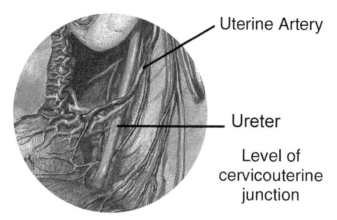

Uterine Artery

Ureter

Level of
cervicouterine
junction

Fig. 8. Uterine arteries and veins, with ureter in view. (*From* Netter: Atlas of Human Anatomy, 5e. Elsevier 2010, plate 383, p. 392.): (Reprinted with permission from Netter Anatomy Illustration Collection, © Elsevier Inc. All Rights Reserved.)

entering this area when performing a hysterectomy, since this surgical area is very vascular (**Fig. 8**).

Passing just underneath and crossing the uterine artery near the cervicouterine junction is the ureter as it travels into the ureteric "tunnel." This area is approximately 2 cm lateral to the side of the cervix and is very near the uterosacral ligament, which is just medial. Therefore, the ureter must be carefully identified during uterine artery ligation/coagulation, any dissection in this area, uterosacral ligament transection, or suture ligation of the uterosacral ligaments. In fact, any transection of the uterosacral ligament may cause subsequent scarring that may pull the ureter medially, closer to the cervix. This situation may make subsequent hysterectomy more likely to injure the ureter. The space just anterior to the base of the cardinal ligament is the paravesical space. The space just posterior (toward the sacrum) is the pararectal space.

Paravesical Space/Paravaginal Space

The paravesical contains the obturator space and is important during pelvic lymph node dissections, as well as reparative vaginal procedures. The paravesical space is a potential space beneath the peritoneum, bordered by the bladder medially, the parietal fascia of the obturator internus muscle laterally, and the base of the cardinal ligament posteriorly. Anteriorly is the pubic bone. Contained within this space is the obturator space. The obturator space is defined from the obliterated umbilical artery medially, to the fascia of the obturator internus muscle laterally, and from the external iliac vein above to the obturator nerve and vessels below. This space contains the obturator nerve, which needs to be identified during pelvic retroperitoneal dissection. As mentioned, this nerve enters the true pelvis at the pelvic brim beneath the iliac veins, and travels on the anterior border of the obturator internus muscle to enter the obturator canal along with the obturator artery and vein. The obturator nerve is actually loosely covered with endopelvic visceral fascia and fatty areolar tissue. During dissection in this area, the nerve is easily exposed by gently sweeping away this tissue. To the reparative vaginal surgeon, this same space is usually approached vaginally through a colpotomy incision and is called the paravaginal space.

Retropubic Space of Retzius

The space of Retzius, or the retropubic space, is a potential avascular space with very vascular borders. The laparoscopist uses this space to perform retropubic urethropexies and paravaginal defect repairs. It consists of an anterior compartment and 2 lateral compartments. The anterior compartment is bounded by the pubic bone anteriorly, and the endopelvic fascial capsule that surrounds the bladder posteriorly. Contained within this endopelvic fascial capsule is the rich network of perivesical venous sinuses within deposits of areolar fat. Centrally over the urethra, just under the pubic arch, is the deep dorsal vein of the clitoris which feeds into these venous channels. Therefore, dissection in the anterior compartment of the space of Retzius must not be directed centrally where these vessels may be lacerated.

The lateral compartment of the space of Retzius (same as the paravesical space) is bounded laterally by the obturator internus fascia and the obturator nerve, artery and vein, just beneath the bony arcuate ridge of the ilium and superior pubic ramus. The posterior border (toward the sacrum) is the endopelvic fascial sheath around the internal iliac artery and vein and its anterior branches, as they course toward the ischial spine. The floor of this lateral compartment is formed by the pubocervical fascia as it inserts into the arcus tendineus fasciae pelvis (fascial white line).

The pubocervical fascia is the thickened anterior portion of the endopelvic visceral fascial (fibromuscular) coat surrounding the vagina. When attached to both fascial white lines laterally and to the cervix posteriorly (anterior portion of the pericervical ring), the pubocervical fascia forms a horizontal platform underneath the bladder. This intact platform prevents anterior vaginal wall prolapse (cystocele). Many cystoceles are caused by a detachment of the pubocervical fascia from one or both fascial white lines, as well as the pericervical ring. This is known as a "paravaginal" defect. Reattachment of this fascial platform to the fascial white lines, as well as the pericervical ring at the level of the ischial spines, is felt to correct this type of cystocele.

The fascial white line (arcus tendineus fasciae pelvis) is a linear thickening of the levator ani fascia from the posterior aspect of the pubic bone in a straight line to the ischial spine. This may be readily seen during a laparoscopic paravaginal defect repair. In the standing female patient, the fascial white line is horizontally oriented. Therefore, in the supine patient, this line travels in an almost vertical manner. Just above the level of the fascial white line may be seen the muscle white line (arcus tendineus levator ani) which is the origin of the levator ani muscles.

When performing a retropubic colposuspension through the laparoscope, the operator must remember that just underneath the external iliac vein and artery is the lateral continuation of the pectineal (Cooper's) ligament on the superior pubic ramus. These structures are hidden in areolar tissue. Therefore, placement of sutures through the pectineal (Cooper's) ligament must stay within 3 to 4 cm of the midline to avoid inadvertent laceration of these great vessels. Accessory obturator arteries and veins are often present. These vessels course from the inferior epigastric vessels and drape across the pectineal (Cooper's) ligament on their way to anastomose with the obturator vessels in the obturator canal. The surgeon must always look for them, because they are often present.

The space of Retzius is easily opened laparoscopically. The peritoneum above the bladder is incised between the obliterated umbilical arteries (medial umbilical folds). The visualization afforded by the magnification of the laparoscope with its bright, directed light source is superb. With dissection in the proper plane, this space can be opened with essentially no blood loss. Excellent exposure to all relevant surgical anatomy is easily obtained. The positive pressure pneumoperitoneum also tamponades small venous bleeders, allowing hemostasis of these vessels to take place.

More inferiorly in the anterior compartment of the space of Retzius, the fatty areolar tissue must be dissected off the anterior vaginal wall to reveal the pubocervical fascia. This is done with a blunt instrument through a laparoscopic port and a finger in the vagina to stabilize the pubocervical fascia. In this area, sutures are placed 2 to 3 cm lateral to the urethrovesical junction in performing a retropubic colposuspension. The urethrovesical junction is identified by the Foley bulb being pulled down gently to the vesical neck. The distal two thirds of the urethra is fused with the anterior vaginal wall. Therefore, sutures placed in the pubocervical fascia and attached to the pectineal (Cooper's) ligament allow significant and sure elevation of the urethrovesical junction close to but not against the pubic bone.

Vesicovaginal Space

The vesicovaginal space is a potential space between the anterior surface of the vagina (pubocervical fascia) and the posterior aspect of the bladder. This space is bordered laterally by the bladder "pillars," which allow for passage of vesical arteries, veins, lymph channels, and visceral nerves, along with the ureters. These structures pass just lateral to the lower uterine segment and cervix, and course on the anterolateral surface of the upper third of the vagina to enter the bladder.

When performing a hysterectomy, the surgeon must incise the uterovesical peritoneal fold. Incising the peritoneal fold and mobilizing the bladder off of the lower uterine segment and the upper portion of the vagina moves the ureters away from the uterine vessels, in addition to moving the bladder to perform the anterior colpotomy incision. The potential vesicovaginal space is created by dissecting avascularly on the pubocervical fascia between the bladder and the cervix and vagina. The extent of dissection depends on the amount of vaginal margin required for suturing the vaginal cuff after the uterus and cervix are surgically excised. Care must be taken not to injure the ureters in the bladder "pillars," which are just lateral and inferior to the edges of the vaginal cuff.

Pararectal Space

The pararectal space is important when performing radical hysterectomies and when excising deep infiltrating endometriosis. This space is easily developed by bluntly dissecting the ureter medially toward the rectum, and by bluntly dissecting laterally to the origin of the uterine artery. The anterior border of this triangular space is the base of the cardinal ligament. The medial border is the ureter dissected toward the rectum, and the lateral border is the internal iliac artery. The space also contains the uterosacral ligament, which is found on the anterior and lateral border as it travels posteriorly toward the sacrum.

Rectovaginal Space

The rectovaginal space is bounded superiorly by the cul-de-sac peritoneum and the uterosacral ligaments, laterally by the iliococcygeus muscles, and inferiorly by the perineal body. Posterior is the endopelvic visceral fascial capsule around the rectum, and anterior is the endopelvic visceral fascial capsule around the vagina. The rectum may be easily and bluntly dissected away from the vagina, since the rectovaginal space is the potential space between these visceral fascial capsules around the rectum and vagina.

Within this space, and just behind the fascial capsule of the vagina, is another endopelvic fascial structure called the rectovaginal septum. The rectovaginal septum attaches to the cul-de-sac peritoneum and the uterosacral ligaments, while inferiorly it attaches directly to the perineal body. Laterally in the upper third of the vagina, the rectovaginal septum attaches to the fascial white lines on the parietal fascia of the levator ani muscles. In the standing female patient, this structure forms an almost horizontal platform between the vagina and rectum and is felt to prevent posterior vaginal wall prolapse (rectocele). Therefore, the reattachment of the rectovaginal septum to the mentioned borders is important in the repair of a rectocele.

SUMMARY

The competent gynecologic surgeon has a sure, working knowledge of the anatomy in the field of pelvic dissection and is expert in the techniques and in the millimeter by millimeter progression of surgical dissections. When operating in the pelvis, the surgeon always asks several questions. The first is, "In what anatomic area am I dissecting?" This question defines the anatomy to be dissected out. The second is, "What dissection techniques will I use here?" The measured steps of surgical dissection give the surgeon the confidence to proceed with the operation, while safeguarding the integrity of the surrounding anatomic structures. With less blood loss and less trauma to the tissues and anatomic structures, the surgeon may expect a better surgical outcome for the patient.

Index

Note: Page numbers of article titles are in **boldface** type.

A

Ablation
  in uterine leiomyoma management, 719–723
Adnexal masses
  diagnosis of, 664–667
    imaging in, 664–665
    laboratory studies in, 665–667
    patient history in, 664
    physical examination in, 664
  in pediatric patients
    laparoscopy for, 766–767
  during pregnancy
    laparoscopy for, 758–759
  presentation of, 663
  prevalence of, 663
  treatment of, 667–673
    laparoscopic management in, **663–676**
    medical therapy in, 667
    surgical, 668–673
      for advanced stage invasive and recurrent ovarian cancer, 671–673
      for benign-appearing lesions, 668–670
      for borderline tumors, 670–671
      for early stage ovarian cancer, 671
      for probable malignancy, 670
Anesthesia/anesthetics
  for laparoscopy during pregnancy, 760
Antiprogestins
  in uterine leiomyomas management, 713
Appendectomy
  during pregnancy
    laparoscopy in, 757–758
Applied Medical port
  in LESS, 745–746
Argon-enhanced electrosurgery, 696
Aromatase inhibitors
  in uterine leiomyomas management, 713
Automatic feedback electrosurgical generators, 694–695

B

Bipolar electrosurgery, 690–691
  ligating-cutting devices in, 691–692

Obstet Gynecol Clin N Am 38 (2011) 789–798
doi:10.1016/S0889-8545(11)00116-1
0889-8545/11/$ – see front matter © 2011 Elsevier Inc. All rights reserved.

obgyn.theclinics.com

United States Postal Service

Statement of Ownership, Management, and Circulation
(All Periodicals Publications Except Requester Publications)

1. Publication Title	2. Publication Number									3. Filing Date
Obstetrics and Gynecology Clinics of North America	0	0	0	-	2	7	6			9/16/11

4. Issue Frequency	5. Number of Issues Published Annually	6. Annual Subscription Price
Mar, Jun, Sep, Dec	4	$275.00

7. Complete Mailing Address of Known Office of Publication (Not printer) (Street, city, county, state, and ZIP+4®)

Elsevier Inc.
360 Park Avenue South
New York, NY 10010-1710

Contact Person: Stephen Bushing

Telephone (Include area code): 215-239-3688

8. Complete Mailing Address of Headquarters or General Business Office of Publisher (Not printer)

Elsevier Inc., 360 Park Avenue South, New York, NY 10010-1710

9. Full Names and Complete Mailing Addresses of Publisher, Editor, and Managing Editor (Do not leave blank)

Publisher (Name and complete mailing address)

Kim Murphy, Elsevier, Inc., 1600 John F. Kennedy Blvd. Suite 1800, Philadelphia, PA 19103-2899

Editor (Name and complete mailing address)

Stephanie Donley, Elsevier, Inc., 1600 John F. Kennedy Blvd. Suite 1800, Philadelphia, PA 19103-2899

Managing Editor (Name and complete mailing address)

Barton Dudlick, Elsevier, Inc., 1600 John F. Kennedy Blvd. Suite 1800, Philadelphia, PA 19103-2899

10. Owner (Do not leave blank. If the publication is owned by a corporation, give the name and address of the corporation immediately followed by the names and addresses of all stockholders owning or holding 1 percent or more of the total amount of stock. If not owned by a corporation, give the names and addresses of the individual owners. If owned by a partnership or other unincorporated firm, give its name and address as well as those of each individual owner. If the publication is published by a nonprofit organization, give its name and address.)

Full Name	Complete Mailing Address
Wholly owned subsidiary of	4520 East-West Highway
Reed/Elsevier, US holdings	Bethesda, MD 20814

11. Known Bondholders, Mortgagees, and Other Security Holders Owning or Holding 1 Percent or More of Total Amount of Bonds, Mortgages, or Other Securities. If none, check box ☐ None

Full Name	Complete Mailing Address
N/A	

12. Tax Status (For completion by nonprofit organizations authorized to mail at nonprofit rates) (Check one)
The purpose, function, and nonprofit status of this organization and the exempt status for federal income tax purposes:
☐ Has Not Changed During Preceding 12 Months
☐ Has Changed During Preceding 12 Months (Publisher must submit explanation of change with this statement)

PS Form 3526, September 2007 (Page 1 of 3 (Instructions Page 3)) PSN 7530-01-000-9931 PRIVACY NOTICE: See our Privacy policy in www.usps.com

---

13. Publication Title	14. Issue Date for Circulation Data Below
Obstetrics and Gynecology Clinics of North America	June 2011

15. Extent and Nature of Circulation		Average No. Copies Each Issue During Preceding 12 Months	No. Copies of Single Issue Published Nearest to Filing Date
a. Total Number of Copies (Net press run)		1441	1450
b. Paid Circulation (By Mail and Outside the Mail)	(1) Mailed Outside-County Paid Subscriptions Stated on PS Form 3541. (Include paid distribution above nominal rate, advertiser's proof copies, and exchange copies)	420	366
	(2) Mailed In-County Paid Subscriptions Stated on PS Form 3541 (Include paid distribution above nominal rate, advertiser's proof copies, and exchange copies)		
	(3) Paid Distribution Outside the Mails Including Sales Through Dealers and Carriers, Street Vendors, Counter Sales, and Other Paid Distribution Outside USPS®	381	290
	(4) Paid Distribution by Other Classes Mailed Through the USPS (e.g. First-Class Mail®)		
c. Total Paid Distribution (Sum of 15b (1), (2), (3), and (4))		801	656
d. Free or Nominal Rate Distribution (By Mail and Outside the Mail)	(1) Free or Nominal Rate Outside-County Copies Included on PS Form 3541	92	75
	(2) Free or Nominal Rate In-County Copies Included on PS Form 3541		
	(3) Free or Nominal Rate Copies Mailed at Other Classes Through the USPS (e.g. First-Class Mail)		
	(4) Free or Nominal Rate Distribution Outside the Mail (Carriers or other means)		
e. Total Free or Nominal Rate Distribution (Sum of 15d (1), (2), (3) and (4)		92	75
f. Total Distribution (Sum of 15c and 15e)		893	731
g. Copies not Distributed (See instructions to publishers #4 (page #3))		548	719
h. Total (Sum of 15f and g)		1441	1450
i. Percent Paid (15c divided by 15f times 100)		89.70%	89.74%

16. Publication of Statement of Ownership

☑ If the publication is a general publication, publication of this statement is required. Will be printed in the December 2011 issue of this publication.   ☐ Publication not required

17. Signature and Title of Editor, Publisher, Business Manager, or Owner	Date
Stephen R. Bushing – Inventory Distribution Coordinator	September 16, 2011

I certify that all information furnished on this form is true and complete. I understand that anyone who furnishes false or misleading information on this form or who omits material or information requested on the form may be subject to criminal sanctions (including fines and imprisonment) and/or civil sanctions (including civil penalties).

PS Form 3526, September 2007 (Page 2 of 3)

Printed and bound by CPI Group (UK) Ltd, Croydon, CR0 4YY

03/10/2024

01040460-0012